TALES FROM
A THOUSAND AND ONE
FREUDIAN NIGHTS

By Janine Baker

Copyright © 2001 by Janine Baker

ISBN 0-7414-0693-4

Cover concept: Janine Baker
Cover design: Christopher A. Master

Published by:

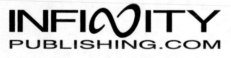

Infinity Publishing.com
519 West Lancaster Avenue
Haverford, PA 19041-1413
Info@buybooksontheweb.com
www.buybooksontheweb.com
Toll-free (877) BUY BOOK
Local Phone (610) 520-2500
Fax (610) 519-0261

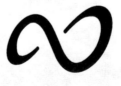

Printed in the United States of America

Printed on Recycled Paper

Published June, 2001

For Dr. Strauss
– there aren't words.

"...We're in no hurry here," psychiatrist trying to be patient. "It'll take us as long as it *takes*...for me to get to know you..." Oh, brother. If that's required for healing, hon, let's wave bye-bye today. How *could* you or anyone know me, my life, my Self? We humans like to talk in linear lies, stringing a false cohesion to the fragments that comprise us. But I am not a story. I am not what I have done. Nor am I a series of feelings because nothing lasts. Something I once cared about means nothing, then wind and rain wash memory onto shore and I'm longing for what I swore I'd never need. And those words, they too, are misleading. A Self is hardly poetry; at best it's graffiti. Scrawled, indiscriminate, selfish. It's our misguided efforts that smash imagery and sound into neat conforming peg holes, to convince ourselves that's how we think. Sequences. Pulses to a single rhythm. An illusion of lunacy helping a world believe it is ordered and sane. *I did this, he did that, she said this, we were there.* And we all agree that yes, that's how it is when Proust nibbles a cookie and yesterdays cascade like leaves. Remembering is no autumn picnic, darling; it's a dynamite keg that splatters and splinters while you pick up an ion or two and try to make sense of it. It's twenty symphonies playing at once and countless loops of film spliced into one another. The mortifying chaos, the delicious freedom of real human thought is a secret well-kept, for no, we are not mad or ever close to it. We are in control, right? I am. Are you? You, too? Okay, cool...good. We're cool. God help us.

I am also my family's memories. Their stories, told and re-told, words so often heard that surely I've lived them. Knowing something means the thinking of it. There are some fantasies I recall with more power than actual experiences. Whether or not we were present when a thing happened ultimately matters less than what it *comes to mean* inside the mind - how we felt, were touched, changed, moved. For that, no real bodies required. So over the years I've taken stories from the lives of those who love me and remolded them into my personal keepsakes, until eventually I remember the *remembering,* and from that I make them mine. It's hardly assault. Any story told is one given away. That's why I wouldn't talk of me for so many years. Ownership, the most prized title. My privacy, a testament that no one could have me.

And now you tell me to talk, to paint a picture of myself to help you see. The mask goes on (I was just chatting while I tied it. See the pretty ribbons that secure it to my head?) And it smiles, this nice mask does, and it charms. It is oh, so responsive. Part mirror, part paper – but no sign of flesh or blood. Don't worry, it promises. You'll like me. Everyone always does.

Captured but cunning, she told her tales to the King,
Every night, she told them.
She told her true and remarkable tales to save her very life.

It feels like I've spent most of my life in bookstores, searching for Me under "Psych" and "Self-Help." In the early 70's it was a total waste of time, save for the ever-present Victor Frankl and a few paperbacks on positive thinking. Eventually *Games People Play* made it to best-seller, somebody screeched a primal scream, and soon Doubleday was stocking texts of Abnormal Psychology. None of it was really about me, but I took any illness I could find.

In the 90's when that icy tip turned glacier, I felt like a damn prophet. Suddenly, Barnes & Noble flaunted 12-step manuals for all things painful. Anxiety and Depression merited their own sections. With the right workbook, we could expect recovery for everything from co-dependency to Satanic abuse, and folks published their self-mutilation, incest and seasonal despair. There were more "Multiples" cranking out autobiographies than most doctors agree even *exist* (let alone have agents).

Mental illness had opened its padded closet.

I ate it up. But in the hundreds of books I bought, there were still few words describing me. Vanilla self-help was written for "regular" functional neurotics, and that blatantly annoyed me. Those people aren't anywhere near sick enough to warrant discussion. Their "issues" (gag) revolve around normal, acceptable lives. Sure, they worry. They fear they're unlovable. They suffer insecurities. But they know they're not insane.

"Please don't worry, honey." My beloved grandmother's signature piece. "You're okay." At seventeen, as I devolved before her very eyes, she was finally willing to consider the possibility of a *physical* problem. "People do get nervous if they don't have enough iron in their blood." So as I imagined things and hid under the kitchen table, holding a thick towel close to my mouth in case I started screaming, my dear grandma (on hands and knees) tried to coax me out with a "good fried liver steak." I loved her so much that I always tried to eat it. "You just don't want anyone to ever think you're 'funny!'" The symptom has not been created that could intimidate her. She saw no need to "do anything" as long as I (with enough calves' liver under my belt) could be propped up and sent into polite society. Secret agents get to carry a cyanide pill just in case. I had my aspirin bottle filled with tranquilizers. *If reality tips, bite down hard and start chewing*. It didn't always work, though, and I often came dangerously close to getting caught. To blowing my cover. To being seen. All the mole wanted was to one day come in from the cold.

"You'll never find yourself in a book." Even two years into it, His Board- Certified Self disapproved of my clinical library. "I've told ya before, everybody's treatment is completely unique."

"But I don't understand what's wrong with me. What my symptoms add up to… Am I psychotic? Or would you even tell me?"

"Yes, I would - and no, you're not. You keep insisting on a label, but I don't *think* in those terms. Diagnoses are for insurance companies – putting people into categories. One short paragraph to sum up a lifetime of conflicts and character traits?"

"I think it would be helpful to me…but if you can't…"

"Look, if I thought you could resist using it as a weapon against yourself, I might be willing to try and squeeze you into some narrow description… but sorry, the answer is no."

"That I wouldn't use it? Or that you'd be willing…"

"Neither!" That irresistible smile. "We can keep going round and round about this, but it's not gonna make me change my mind."

"Or mine."

"Oh, I know that." Stalemate? I should be so lucky. He leaned towards me wearing his *but seriously though, folks…* expression. "There's such an irony here – because the *root* of your symptoms – oh, that's in plenty of books. In thousands - novels, poems - it's been written about for centuries -- love and loss and aggression and loneliness -- the human *condition*. And the trouble you cause yourself comes from hiding from it - pretending for so long that you don't have ordinary human needs." I just stare at him, hearing it all, rejecting it all, devastated at being misunderstood. "Now that might not be the 'diagnosis' you're looking for, but it's true!" No one could actually be charmed by that obnoxious, self-satisfied smile.

Prelude

Yet, when he looks at me, I melt.

His head cocked to one side, eyes dancing.

He has become every cliché.

Waiting for him, I secretly open my compact, keeping it inside my purse, glancing down, checking make-up, smoothing bangs. I've turned into a forty-year old teenager.

He touches my hand. Heat through my body until against better judgment,

I feel a smile – one I didn't even plan. Not a Born-To-Charm smile or I'll-Get-'Em With-*This*-Look, but a real one that broke through all by itself. Almost shy. A little hesitant. Filled with hope. I've become what I spent my life ridiculing.

It can't last. There is comfort in that.

But still…

There is no one else like this man. And he knows - knows I've let none in my bed. Knows I grow tired of everything, can feel a lifetime in minutes… no. I used to. This desire has lasted from its first moments through the night our bodies touch. And without hating. Not hurting. Sustained. Over time. The world is upside down.

Feeling his hair, his back. Literally loving what I touch. Even while knowing what it is. Just the flesh of an ordinary man.

And my brain searches for some map of how I got here, to this place that is not me.

The Custom House ?

okay, okay...
Part One

My life has been hard to start. Wait, rewind that. In truth, beginnings are no challenge at all. In fact, they're my specialty. Forty years of nothing but "First Acts" and my favorite hobby is still to shake my life from side to side like a giant cosmic Etch-a-Sketch, and make yesterday's words and plans vanish before everyone's eyes. Should anybody pester me too much about that now obsolete picture, I just walk away from said person and *really* start fresh. Small loss, ultimately. Nothing is forever. Besides, there is little in this world more beautiful than a completely blank screen.

From here on - things change! This is the day my _real_ self is born!

Remember last year when I foolishly proclaimed "NOW I'm here for _real_?" Well, just forget that, cause it's clear that _today_ is my _true_ turnaround.

*All those times I've said "This Is The Moment"... I finally realize there's no such thing! And today – the day I realized **that** – is the start of my life finally being different!*

Oh, brother.

My personal fragrance would be called "Potential." The-girl-most-likely-to/ wonder-why-she-never-*does*. (Hey, give me a break, guys. I am, after all, a little nuts. In spite of my grandmother's frantic P.R. campaign, I insist on being described in those questionable terms).

The world tilts. No one sane could understand. Reality is not a "state," it's only a thought. Life itself changes colors and scenes of my daily existence suddenly look like they're being directed by a different film-maker – with avant garde, surrealistic lighting. What seemed like a happy little comedy can instantly become a Scorsese film. An ordinary drama turns into the Twilight Zone, precipitated by nothing but a blink, a breath, by absolutely nothing except the passing of an instant. The world alters on a dime. The physical stage remains, the actors are the same *people*, but the look of everything - the feel, its grain, the tone and texture of all I see and hear has become surreal. The gods, if They're there, are playing with Einstein's laws, and like a dream, exactly like a Dream, all bets of Time and Space are off. Reality is *not fixed*, never was or will be. No one sees that, can't let themselves see. One quiver of a kaleidoscope and Alice flies to the other side of her mirror. This is the world you want me to inhabit, to live and care in? Others just watch little Alice and expect her to keep playing as if nothing's happened. "Let's take a little walk outside..." As if the World is there.

I've seen a few therapists. Off and on. Their pills help me cope. None of their words have made a dent. And now, after ten years of surviving unofficially on my uncle's secret valium, I'm off to greet another one. Little choice. Time to make a new friend. Walking from the subway, I turn onto his street and review my opening lines. In and out of this spot called Sanity. Extreme anxiety states unrelenting for days on end. Feelings of not being real, of being dead. Of not having a Self at all.

Dr. Alexander Strauss. A referral from The Payne Whitney Clinic. Casey was surprised I didn't want her therapist to suggest someone. Keeping all neuroses in the family, I guess. Thanks, babe. I'll just get out the Yellow Pages and handle matters with some poor unsuspecting stranger. Blanche DuBois knew best.

"Panic attacks..." according to magazines of Normal People "...affect many highly successful individuals." Yeah sure, we can call it that for awhile. Let's pretend.

Of course, I am far from what anyone would call "successful," 35 years old, 163 I.Q. and the not-so-proud owner of a not-so-illustrious career as a word processing temp. There are parts of myself I understand in a way most people do not. There are things I know about myself, about the world at large that most people will never comprehend. I'll stop with that now, because there's no need to tease. There are things about myself I will never share. In the end, I'll be vindicated either because things were as I suspected and it's safer to be the only one who knows – or because I was merely going insane all along and who the hell needs witnesses for that one?

Somebody's face reflects from a car window. Mine, my face, whosoever that is. I look so much like them, my family. Small features, pale skin, baby fine hair, high forehead. Never had a shot at believing an "adoption fantasy." I am of them. Or *am* them. Looking into any mirror, it's *their* eyes staring back, as if looking for themselves. Then come the words, my mother rambling about who I looked like – never her, not some relative. Movie stars. The people who lived on her walls.

My past is a paradox, not much more than dust-covered boxes, but still fresh as odorless eggs. I wake up every day begging to finally be rid of its mark.

Ideal life: to be an amnesiac.

Logical Syllogism 149: Hating everything I've done, Ergo...I hate who I am.

I'm only happy when I forget I exist. Watching other people's lives. In and out. Visit and leave. Sample, not gluttony. And no after-taste.

As I walk into the new doctor's lobby, somebody whispers "help me." Please help me keep my front just a little while longer. No pretense can last forever. Things have been unraveling so fast as of late. Working will be my downfall...the days in and out...days with the same faces. Hours of confinement and servitude. "But you're making a decent hourly, now!" Casey beamed with my last temp assignment. I'm a goddamn secretary. It's okay. But it is. It won't be much longer. Whenever the jig's up, it will be a relief in a way. No more games. No more trying. As I ring his doorbell, I feel like I've shown up to turn myself in. He sounded like such a decent person over the phone. Here I am, doctor. Lock me up when the time comes, and please don't let anyone hurt me.

He's casual, but well dressed in a gray turtleneck, dark jacket and slacks. But it's that impeccable office that really gets me. Large burgundy and indigo chairs, oak bookcases, an Oriental rug, wrought-iron floor lamps, a Monet print, some Egyptian bookends. Eclectic but every single color offset to a perfect palette. "My God," I say and hate that those were my first words. "It's like a therapist's office from the movies!"

"Which movie?" He asks.

"No, none in particular." I hate even more that he didn't understand. "I just meant the Hollywood ideal, central casting, you know. It's… perfect!" A slight smile, appropriately careful, and that's certainly a good way to be with me. "Of course," I just can't shut up. "what do they say? Looks can be deceiving, huh?"

"Well," he chuckles, loosening up as we sit. "That was a lot of information there." Now it's a much better smile. Have we decided already that I'm not insane? Similar mistakes have proved costly.

Three sessions right off the bat, that's his trip. We agree to see each other three times this week, and after that, decide if we want to work together. Interesting. That's a lot of information about *him*, too. Money don't do it for ya, huh? No one can just buy their way into your arms. Instead, you hold a 150-minute audition. Piece of cake. For my first monologue, I've chosen a dramatic recitation from one of the classic tragedies…

The terror of my anxiety. Years of seeing a psychiatrist when I was a teenager – and that is definitely the correct verb. I merely showed up every week, said I was still petrified and let him reassure me that I wasn't necessarily turning into my mother. The crazy woman. The woman I detest, resist and condemn to anyone who listens. But in secret, one of many I will take to my grave, sometimes her paranoid delusions make sense to me. I call her mad. Silently, I suspect she's right. Folie a deux? Or just similar chemistries. I took daily medications for over 20 years. Valium, stellazine, elavil, mellaril. Got better for awhile, and then it'd come back. With a vengeance. Don't wish "getting better" on me. I couldn't survive it. "Degenerative psychosis." I'm very well-read, so don't try to protect me from facts. And don't be fooled just because I'm crazy enough to act sane – any normal person who felt like this wouldn't attempt to go to school, or work, wouldn't dare try to hide so much. Never held a regular job for longer than a year. Well, not entirely true. Ready for a little shock therapy? There was my seven year stint in the sex trade industry. (Not even a blink, doc? Not bad). It wasn't prostitution. Well, *legally* not. I acted out fantasies with male clients. Dominance and submission, role playing, you-name-it with props and costumes, no actual intercourse, but nearly anything else. It was hideous, but I had to get by. I don't look the type, right? Listen up, boy. I am no type at all - because nothing visible is remotely *me*. When my mind gets that way, I can't keep up a

5

schedule and can't work nine to five. I'm sorry. It's too much for anybody to understand. It's no one's fault they can't help."

Your face is so gentle, sympathetic. (Ya didn't really hear that, I guess. My prediction that you'll be flaccid with me? That in spite of all good intentions, you won't be able to get your professional Dick to even twitch). "I sit here talking and I seem normal, but no one sees…"

"Whatever *normal* is…" Oh, please don't be a jerk so soon. What you don't know is how different I am underneath all sensory evidence. How sweet, how responsive I appear. I am the queen of response. And most of you make me sick. By the way, no children, no lover. Ever. Never had a boyfriend, no desire to change it. Romance and couples are stuff Other People care about - and I spend my life not understanding why anyone cares about the things they do. I'm not like other people, and what a glorious world it would be if everyone around me could accept that. Maybe I understand the scientists best. Obsessions with time and space. Interests that do not include their own bodies. "Did you study the Sciences?" No. Not formally. "How come?" Not interested. My ambitions include being able to sleep and not be terrorized by dreams. I hope one day I can look in a mirror without danger – trust that everything in reality won't become reverse-imaged for days or longer. To not hear thoughts that whisper secrets about when I'll go mad, and how this world is not what it seems. It's been like this off and on for twenty years. I had a college scholarship but left after two months. Severe breakdown at 18, and that's the state I fear is coming back. Yes, I work now. I can seem normal. Stay tuned. It won't last. I have friends, not a problem area. One best friend whom I adore. My lover? No. I love her more than that. I sacrifice for her, I give TO her. She's more important than desire, her talent, her abilities…Casey's an actress, see, and there's more to that, okay? I supported her for years, I believe in her career, she's going to be a star. I invested in her, we were roommates. I paid all the rent. You don't understand, I see you don't… I helped her out with money while she took classes and did showcases. We're the best of friends, I know it sounds like why would I support her, but it's what I wanted to do. Other people don't get it – what else is new? She's the good in my life, she and my grandmother. They matter. She just got engaged, Casey did. And I know they can't be here forever, but for as long as they are, I need to be okay. A little secret? I wouldn't exist without them. Won't. It'll end then.

"Literally?" I don't know.

Last week I couldn't leave the house. I thought the Revealing was close. The End of all ends where I'd finally be unable to kid myself anymore. Images bleeding into each other, faces looked odd. I wasn't even sure it was really Casey. She thought I had the flu, that's what I told her. She doesn't know how bad things get, knows I get anxious, but doesn't realize what could happen. And she shouldn't have to know. I call my grandmother when I'm feeling my worst...there's no one else I'd talk to that way...she's old, did I say that? She is, getting old... It's happening soon and there is nothing to be done.

The doctor's expression is dear. Furrowed brow, sympathetic eyes. Leaning forward, listening carefully. He is visibly touched. *Thank you, thank you. Now lest ya think I'm just too depressing to deal with, I will now do my Comic Piece...*

Let me simply describe The Family. Trust me, humor will flow. It's an odd little play – my childhood. There's only one set – the inside of our house. We tried hard to never leave. First there's Cleo, my grandmother. Matriarch Extraordinaire. But that title implies Southern airs of nobility which we certainly were not. Cleo is goddess-on-a-budget with her dime-store aprons and felt house slippers, fighting off bill collectors (or trying to seduce them with home-made pie in lieu of anything spendable). In my life she is without question the Glue Holding Earth Together. In fact, the other actors in this play rarely speak to each other. They talk only to Cleo – constantly and especially with complaints. "He hurt my feelings." "She's acting like she might not go to work today." "I think he has beer – go say something..." Because of the size and scope of her role, she never leaves the stage. As this is such a demanding part, it requires an actress of super-human endurance and mythic motivation. The only reward is knowing that without her, the entire play and its characters would cease to exist. The Support-less Cast: Mary Jane and Otis. My mother and uncle. (Cleo's grown children who never got around to leaving home). She - a high functioning schizophrenic. He - a low functioning alcoholic. Given those facts, the two actors don't really need a script. Just let them improvise freely around the maypole that is their mother.

7

And I, ah, I was the child queen who literally ran the house. They let a five-year old scared little kid decide what to eat for dinner, what time to go to bed, where we should all sit to watch TV. My grandmother tells the story that one night in the rain, a wild New Orleans thunderstorm, she and I were running for a bus till I stopped in my tracks and started to cry. Scared to get on, I said I didn't like how the bus looked, and cried and begged till we walked home, 12 blocks in a cold night storm. "Well, honey, you didn't want to get on. You always did have a mind of your own." I was three. My grandmother would do anything for me. Has and will. I'm embarrassed at how much they worship me, but especially her, at the things I've gotten her to do.

Harmless, But Odd Factoids: Otis is chronically worried that the neighbors are too curious. In prevention mode, he puts scotch tape on all 19 window shades, sticking every inch of them to the inevitably peeling woodwork. The telephone (that other dangerous link to La Monde) is kept in a thick cardboard box with three fluffy pillows mashed on top to muffle that jarring ring. He's convinced the only callers could be bill collectors or some fringe relative (or one of the dreaded neighbors checking to see who's home). If any of us are out of the house, he does remove the top two pillows so he stands a chance of hearing the phone ("in case I'm needed in emergency"), but adds extra tape to the shades. Bear in mind, this drama takes place in New Orleans, and since our heroes can't afford air conditioning, the crypt is well, a bit humid. By mid-summer, we'd make a few concessions like turning on a kitchen window fan and reluctantly opening the front door. For six hours at a time, Otis would sit on the porch. Just sit. Cleo brought him beers, and thanked him for looking out for us. Mary Jane would pace and quietly panic because he might "say something" to someone walking by. I was staked out in the living room, watching him watching them. It was a tight little outfit, our brigade, and we did damn good. No other soldiers ever found our bunker.

Through every day and night, they doted on me. I am what happens to children who never hear "No." People are dangerous – well, that was the press. Others (out there) are vile, sneaky and mean. Sadistic men with their sex obsessions. Women who betray their own. We were the "good guys" - I merely shuddered to imagine the Others.

We did as we chose, my mother, my uncle and I. With Cleo as ringmaster, the inmates ran the circus. That's not a "loosening of association," doctor; I was mixing metaphors. The Powerful Grandmother's only admonition was to keep our world inside that house. "You wouldn't ever want people to think we're funny…" Oh, my darling. They couldn't have thought we were any funnier if we wore polka dot pants and threw buckets of confetti.

The doctor is chuckling now. Pretty hard. So I sit back with an awkward smile and run my hand through my hair. First Rule of Comedy – always end the set on a really big laugh.

More stories poured out, offering promise. Night after another, Scheherazade filled his mind, leaving him pleased - but never sated.

By the end of our third trial session ("Hold on! It's a *consultation*" he laughs. "No one's on trial here!") Then he offers "I'd like to try and help ya." That gentle smile. I want to keep him, this kind man who seems to like me. "You could probably limp along with tranquilizers, but if we do some work together I bet you can have a lot more." Okay, now *you* hold on. You actually believe I could survive with just drugs? Hell, maybe that should be my option. In fact, it's the best damn prognosis I've ever gotten. Then I realize. Of course, he's optimistic. He doesn't know me.

"Okay, great." I beam. "Let's give it a try." He nods. Poor idiot. Just get out that prescription pad, hon. Do what you ya do best.

Monday 6:00 p.m. A mere three weeks later.

Without understanding why, I feel remarkably better. In 22 days this man has actually made a difference. We've talked about my mother's schizophrenia, and he seems to understand. The madness in genes, neurological weakness. What I am/was/will be. What it was to be with her. Her touch. Her looks. I despised the way she wanted me, as if loving *me* was the cause of all the pain. "It *can* be hard on a schizophrenic when she loves…those intense feelings can be way too much to handle…" I tell him over and over more than he needs to hear, but when he seems to understand, it's catnip and I need to tell more. "Some children of psychotic parents…" He is, just maybe, not afraid to see. I explain a little about the movies, the gruesome ones. We shouldn't have gone, neither she nor I, but we had to – we liked going every single week and sometimes there was nothing else playing. It was no one's fault that we had to watch what was there. She was no mother at all to show me those faces. Burned into my mind. Hers, too, yes I know, but I am my own keeper of blood and evil. Getting medicine is no problem now. He sees why I need it. What I need most is a place to finally put the stories, the mouth of a dragon perhaps…to take my histories and eat them or burn them, and never give them back.

Memory. 10 years old.

Blue light from an old black and white television set. The smells of beer and fried fish, a tingling of pans, clanging of a dropped fork. Cleo bustles in the kitchen, has gone to get catsup for him and tries to sneak in a few minutes of dishwashing on the side.

"No, Mama!" Otis hollers. "I *told* ya, I will clean up!"

"Oh, I know, honey! I just put a skillet in the sink." He's calm tonight although there's beer and she'll do anything to keep that peace. Later he'll be too tired to make good on his offer, and how bad he'll feel if he thinks he failed her.

Otis and Mary Jane, two blue-lit silhouettes – and they *are* only that. Images. Reflections of who they might have been. I feel Knowledge coming, and as always, it will be more than I want to know. *The Twilight Zone* is my news program because I am convinced there are Truths told there. *Oh, those are just silly spooky stories...* Okay. But unlike most kids, I understand the secret code. I know why they tell us fairy tales and ghost stories, and I know why adults jump when the shocking revelation is made at the end of science fictions. It's preparation. A warning in sheep's clothing. The world is not what it appears, but to come forward and say so would drive children insane. Instead they prep us, tease us, lay breadcrumbs to lead us...and maybe by the time we figure it out, by the time we face the terror, just maybe we can survive the knowing. I saw something on the moon last night.

In the last few minutes *The Twilight Zone* episode reveals that nothing is real after all. On *The Outer Limits*, a scene in a living room with pretty gray carpet and soft speaking people, till across the floor moves a dismembered hand... a normal looking scene, normal as can be. That's when nightmares move in. *Lots of kids have bad dreams.*

It's in The Bible, you know. Eve's apple is a hint. Plain as day, loud as sound. Even god felt a pang of compassion and warned us in print. His tree of Knowledge holds the secret truth - *Knowing* is our hell. Blissful till then. Until we saw. More than we could stand.

There's no such thing as flying saucers, but people keep seeing them, and no one believes but everyone talks and no one,

11

NO one knows who's one of them, and who's of us. There are truths told on Otis' special radio. "The things they don't want everybody to know…" Wide band.

I saw something on the moon last night, and I know that I have changed. It was not a cloud or a reflection or any of the lies. I stared right at it and it saw me back. It knows I know. *All children believe in ghosts and monsters.* But in the light of day, they can stop. My mind is a plaything that plays with *me.*

The room moves in its blue light. Mary Jane laughs at Ralph Kramden and I look at her and smile. I can see in her eyes that she thinks more than she says. Something has already driven her mad, and I have no idea if she has the strength not to tell. Out of the corner of my eye, I catch movement inside her chair. Things do move, things unseen. They could. They might. It happens in dreams. My breathing is too slow. Fingernails into my foot, so carefully, not to bleed just to help. The chair could be alive, and I won't ever say it out loud, okay, okay, never, never out loud. My hand onto Cleo's lap. Help me. Hold me. She touches my head. Nothing helps. Even she is powerless. *All children think up scary things. Kids are like that. Some little girls have overactive imaginations.* It was never this bad until I looked to the moon. Life will be divided now between the days before this and the hell to follow. The fate of a child ruptured because on the wrong day at the wrong minute, she made a poor choice. There will come a time when everyone will face it. When flocks are brought together, possibly for slaughter, as one never really knows. The killer is this – I know I'm only imagining. I know what's real. I think I do. Or no one does.

You'll outgrow it.

When?

Every year after that, I learn a little more. Wishing I could forget, then slowly trying to face that this was the beginning of true madness. Whatever I imagine takes on a life of its own. There is no Stop button for me. By fifteen I've read of schizophrenia and how it starts and when it starts and in whom it starts. And finally I understand. No, I am not really insane. I just might as well be.

School was so hard. Not the learning part, the showing up. It was all just too much, too many people, too many words, too much intensity. Not every child is meant to interact. "I hated it too, honey," dear Cleo nodded. "I just don't know what to tell you. They make you go. You have to go." My face must have hurt her. "Just go today, and then I'll see what I can do." In retrospect, was she actually imagining she could get me out of the whole thing? The woman whose sincerity was equaled only by her gall. Excessive absences in grades 1-3 finally brought me face-to-face with the school social worker, Miss Gardner. She was going to talk to me. That was all. She was going to talk. We were going to just talk. That was all. As if that wasn't unbearable unto itself. I never told Cleo, because it was clear they thought something was wrong with me. They were trying to do something. They were after me. They knew.

"Do you like your class, Janine?" Miss Gardner asked too much. When she had trouble getting answers, she finally let me talk about whatever I chose. A neighbor's cat had just had kittens, and that seemed a safe topic. Once a week, for half an hour, we chatted, and I only wondered how much longer I'd be allowed to live. I was terrified of running out of material. In the end ol' Miss Gardner proved to be very helpful (just not in the way she'd hoped). For such a frightened little mess, I realized I was doing a damn good job of evading the woman. As she got bolder in efforts to win my friendship, I had my first experience of feeling competent. I appeared to slowly open up, my words sounding less guarded, until I even confessed to getting scared when I had to talk in class. I added that it's too bad about me having to miss so much school and was worried that other kids didn't understand what it was like having chronic "bronchitis." (Didn't want to sound precocious).

"Bronchitis," she corrected with a warm smile. I grinned back and said "thank you." She clearly liked me. And trusted me. My work there was done.

Monday 5:45 p.m.

"You and Casey are roommates?" Strauss asks. Okay, I guess he's right. I really *don't* talk about my present life very much.

"No, not now," I say with enormous neutrality. "We used to be. For years. But last May, that's when she got engaged." After years of diligent failure, she's found him - and secretly I hoped he'd be another let down. No, I'm not proud of that. So I gave them the apartment as a wedding present, and that's where they live, together now, in our house; well that's what she wanted...they were looking and I realized I could move easier...Casey is the one with all the furniture...

"A pretty big wedding gift." I hear ya. And I've said it before, babe. No one understands me and Casey.

I'm kinda strange, her friends tell her.

I'm too generous, they secretly tell me.

We must be lovers, they tell each other.

They envy us, they tell no one.

She gives back, and that's the part no one gets. I needed a lottery to play, and a chance to survive. When she makes it, when she's a star, maybe just maybe they'll see.

"You like the new doctor?" she asked last night, and I'm sure I gave some acceptable answer. Responding in a way that makes her feel we're alike, or at least that I'm comprehensible. That's what answers are. In all conversations, someone speaks till I reply, and we saunter around as I find a way to help them be okay about us. Casey has been in her own share of therapy rooms where she's complained about men and how hard things are in show business. She works on building self-esteem and learning to state her needs and from it all, as I listen and encourage, I realize that I have a normal friend. In that statement is my solace. Playing Rhoda to her Mary is the oasis from what I know myself to really be. She buys it, too, this brilliant sophisticated woman. And the guilt there could fill twenty sessions.

Hard bein' so easy...

6:30 p.m. Thursday

Dr. Strauss' **waiting** room. (Excellent name for it)

Twice a week I keep showing up five minutes early (and consistently, he's about seven minutes late). It's really okay. This is something I can offer – to wait quietly, lacking any urgent place

14

to be. His other patients with their tightly wired little schedules probably flinch over a five-minute transgression. Being different, I give my doctor a break. I can do that much. What I *cannot* seem to do is get better, and for that I hope he forgives me. I'm not a bad patient. Punctual, appreciative, attentive. I've tried damned hard to be this easy to deal with.

"Do you think he's helping you?" Casey asked this morning.

"Does talking to that psychiatrist seem to help?" Cleo asked when I was 18.

"Do you think it helps when you can talk to the social worker?" That was my fourth grade teacher.

"Not really, Miss Bartchey," I said quietly, eyes darting from the chalkboard to the floor. "I'm sorry."

Every Sunday I belonged to my mother. It was our movie day and "She *lives* for it, honey. That is what's keeping her alive." (quote from **The Declarations of Cleo-dependence**). Sometimes we saw kiddy movies with bright colors and songs and beautiful animals and charming children. Other times, we took the bus downtown to darkly brood with the likes of Bette Davis, Geraldine Page and Paul Newman. Adult Stories packed with desire, revenge, sex and death. *Mary Poppins, On The Beach, Thomasina, Whatever Happened To Baby Jane?* We saw a picture about a little girl who befriended a lion, and we saw one where a man was decapitated. It seems a jealous lover with a big hatchet can be more trouble than Safari animals. The sounds of screaming when a woman was disemboweled just wouldn't go away. Granted, I never actually said "super-califragilistic-expialidocious," but then it's a silly word from a stupid movie, and we all know movies aren't real. My mother is sick, and no one thought to keep us apart.

One day Cleo had to come get me at school because I couldn't tell if I was dreaming. My face buried in her apron, I was safe. Smells of onion and potatoes, damp strong hands that literally held my blood inside its skin. But even that couldn't last. In a few years, nothing would comfort because even Cleo's hands were flawed. She'd still touch me, always, always touch, but in place of her strength I started feeling frailty. And I kept watch for the weakening. This god who could also die. No one told me that, never told me or gave me a running chance - before I started needing. I began mourning her thirty years ago.

Lately, I've started thinking that maybe Strauss sees. This doctor could be one of the good ones, able to appreciate the kind of upbringing I went through. Sees what they did. All 3 of them. Not that I'm saying I'm better, oh no. We're crazy, every last one of us.

And then today, I walk over to the chair. Like any other day. No one knows what's coming. Ever.

"They *made* ya crazy, huh?" His smile looked forced.

"My mother and uncle did, yes. They didn't mean to, I realize that."

"And what if I said 'you're just *not*...not crazy at all...'" Then I'd say you *are* them, seeing only what you want to see. And I've had no fucking idea what this process is really about.

Monday 6 p.m. session.

"Of *course* I'm hyper vigilant," I try to chuckle. "My whole life, Cleo and my mother, they never took their eyes off of me. My every breath, every move... it'd make anybody this way..." Pauses. So many of them lately. "I'm sorry, I guess there aren't words for it."

"Then we'll find words." My, aren't you speedy. No matter how much I appreciate your determination, the message is misplaced. Words do not always clarify. Often they're only filling up a room to stop things from being heard. "They're all we have..."

Very unfortunate. Anyone can talk. Toddlers and lunatics ramble incessantly without stopping to breathe. It's not communication at all, instead only the search for a sound, a ping of gibberish to accent their little one-person show. Utterances in a cartoon of Follow The Bouncing Ball, punctuating notes on the scale of their emotions. Nothing more than filler noise. Background singing. Sounds to keep truth at bay.

I should know. Every second of every inch of every space in our house, there were words. "They're all talkers, huh?" I'll go again. Every second of every day in every room in every breath…there were words. Sometimes at school, we were told to sit and read. Twenty kids and one adult in a wordless room. Just breathing and blood flowing with hearts pumping, a cough, a sneeze, only bodies. In silence. And it was absolutely terrifying.

Waiting For BillyJoe

(An awful little play with no intermission)

Softly under the dialogue, Bobbie Gentry sings…

MARY JANE
It worries me to hear that part.

OTIS
It's just a *song*, Mary Jane!

MARY JANE
I like them when they're not on the bridge.

CLEO
I thought the whole song was up on that bridge.

OTIS
That's right, Mama. At least you *listen*…

MARY JANE
They were young and in love.

OTIS
Yeah, that's what killed him.

MARY JANE
He was wrong to do that. I admit it. Even if she broke his heart.

OTIS
It doesn't say nothin' about her breaking his heart!

CLEO
No, I bet they were happy together.

MARY JANE
Maybe she wrote him a Dear John letter. That's what they threw off the bridge.

OTIS
For cryin' out loud, Mary Jane, they didn't throw any letter, Mary Jane! Where's your brain? It was a baby!

CLEO
Otis, honey, don't say that…

MARY JANE
Nobody'd throw a little baby off a bridge.

OTIS
It wasn't alive, for cryin' out loud! They got together and she had his baby…

MARY JANE
He put it in her, and she got knocked up and …

CLEO
Otis, please.

OTIS
I'm not sayin' he didn't love her. But they were kids, and maybe she got an abortion or the baby was born dead. They had to get rid of the evidence.

MARY JANE
It could've been a letter from *him* – saying he'd done her wrong…

OTIS
Like your boyfriend Teddy Kennedy! He got rid of the evidence!

CLEO
They said he was going to talk tonight. Don't you want to see him on T.V., Mary Jane?

MARY JANE
Nobody cares about him. That's what wrong. He made them all jealous.

OTIS
He ran, you know. Sunk her and ran.

MARY JANE
He says it was a bad accident.

CLEO
He didn't mean to drive off the bridge...

OTIS
I've always said it - water is very dangerous.

CLEO
You should never go near a lake at night.

OTIS
At least Billy Joe killed himself. He didn't take it out on anybody else.

MARY JANE
He wasn't a politician!

CLEO
No, he was a simple boy. The whole thing is so sad.

MARY JANE
That Bobby Gentry didn't have to write that song. The green eyes of the monster.
When they all get jealous....

CLEO
Remember how jealous your boyfriends used to get. Especially Monty Ratner.

MARY JANE
But he wasn't like this. This is a mean jealous where they don't want him to have anything. They hate him.

CLEO
I guess that's more envy then.

MARY JANE
All right. It's envy.

CLEO
You're never like that. You're always glad for people to be happy.

MARY JANE
Well, yes. I try to be. I feel so bad if someone is in a bad way like Teddy is now. He doesn't deserve this.

OTIS
Are you still talking about him?

MARY JANE
Honey, this is important to her.

OTIS
He got himself in trouble; that's all. He got caught. See, he didn't have an "out." Three things you need for any job: an angle, a system, and an out. He had the angle. Now we don't know if he planned it or not, but either way he had the reason to do it. And he had a system. It wasn't a very good system though. He didn't think his system through enough. But that wouldn't have mattered if he'd had an out. But he didn't. So he got caught.

MARY JANE
Don't talk like that. Ted didn't want to hurt anybody.

OTIS

Well, he sure didn't help her! He could've gone into the water and pulled her up. She wouldn't have been dead. He could've pulled her right out. But he stalled. Now why would he stall if it wasn't part of his system?

MARY JANE

I sure care about him. I pray for him every night.

CLEO

When is he going to talk to us?

OTIS

At 8:00 they said.

CLEO

Do you think she was his girlfriend? She probably was I guess.

MARY JANE

She was his whore. I'd be his little whore and let him stick it in me day or night.

CLEO

No, honey, you'd be his girlfriend.

MARY JANE

That's what I mean. It's not the end of the world for a man to have a girlfriend on the side sometimes. She was young too, and blonde. That made more people jealous.

OTIS

You always like the blondes! Always thought Jean Harlow, Lana Turner, Betty Grable were better than the other ones.

MARY JANE

The blondes all have something. Everybody secretly knows that.

OTIS

I never did. I think Hedy Lamarr, Vivian Leigh...

MARY JANE

All right. Vivian Leigh in Gone With The Wind had "IT".
She did. But she was unusual. You have to admit that.

OTIS

All the good movie stars are dead anyway.

MARY JANE

Don't say that.

OTIS

But she didn't *need* to be a blonde is all I'm trying to say.

MARY JANE

Well, nobody needs to be a blonde. I just think they have
more is all.

CLEO

You always looked wonderful as a blonde. Everyone thought
so.

OTIS

Yes, yes you did. In your day, you looked good.

MARY JANE

But I couldn't find the right kind of man. Never anybody like
Teddy.

OTIS

Well, he just killed one blonde…

MARY JANE

That's stupid talk. I don't want to hear anything like that.

CLEO

We have to remember how much he means to her. No reason
to talk that way if it hurts her.

MARY JANE

You don't believe that, too, do you, Mama? You don't
believe he hurt her.

CLEO
No. I don't think so. I wouldn't want to think that.

OTIS
See, that's the funny thing about you. You don't want to
think something, so you don't think it. That must be pretty good.

CLEO
I think it's a good way to be.

MARY JANE
He's going to talk to us at 8:00.

CLEO
Do you want to go in the front room and turn on the TV?

MARY JANE
I wish he was the president. I'm gonna pray for him to be our
president.

OTIS
That's over with now. He sunk that dream in the
Chappaquidick!

MARY JANE
He can be anything he wants to be. I wish he wanted to
marry me. That's what I wish. I would be faithful to him. You
know I would.

CLEO
Of course you would.

MARY JANE
I would. I hope he'd know that.

CLEO
Sure. He'd trust you. He'd know how much you love him.

MARY JANE
All the bad things that can happen.

CLEO
Let's don't dwell on it ...

MARY JANE
Like the movie stars' children.   Some of them commit suicide. I always pray that more won't.

OTIS
Praying doesn' have anything to do with anything.

CLEO
Oh, I think it does.

MARY JANE
Maybe not enough of us pray. That's why Teddy is in so much trouble now.

CLEO
Well, we'll say a prayer for him tonight. We always do.

OTIS
I'm not an atheist, you know that. I am an agnostic. An agnostic says "I don't KNOW if there is a god or if there isn't." So I'm an agnostic.

MARY JANE
I wish you'd pray.

CLEO
Oh, he believes, I think.

OTIS
Why do you say that?!   Didn't I just tell you for the hundredth time I am an agnostic?

CLEO
Okay, okay, you are then.

OTIS

You just don't like to argue, Mama. You get too nervous.

CLEO

Well, that may be true.

OTIS

And it's not even real war. There's a difference you know. They called it the Korean CONFLICT because no one declared war.

CLEO

But it's better to all get along, don't you think?

OTIS

Of course. That's the best, yes. If it can be done. But living here, in this city where you can't even go out for a walk without people staring at you... it's enough to make anybody have trouble.

CLEO

We won't always live here.

MARY JANE

I don't want to go anywhere. I want us all to stay right here. Tight and up right....

CLEO

We're not going anywhere at all. We're just talking. Janine, honey stay over here...come sit here by me.

Cleo's eyes are warm spotlights that never leave my face. At Mary Jane and Otis' most ridiculous comments, she smiles, then winks. At me. She and I see it, only she and I. They're idiots and she has to tolerate them. I am the only one she loves.

OTIS

Look, Mary Jane, I made a paper airplane to show you. Now watch, you have got to understand. Paper wouldn't fall off a bridge! Now watch and you'll learn somethin'...

25

Dear Miss Bartchey,

Please excuse Janine for not having her homework. The Ode To Billy Joe was on the radio last night.

Maybe that's why I'm always imagining sentences, remembering words…(we try hard in my family not to actually say "hearing voices"). When I'm feeling sane I marvel at the purity of sounds. A fan whirs, a window shade flaps – and those noises are nothing except what they are. There is no hidden message if played backwards, and no subliminal voice embedded within the ordinary sounds. "Imaginary voices" are hard to describe. Even psychiatric definitions get it wrong as much as right. "…delusional perception of words, commands or messages in the absence of real external stimuli." That's not true, at least for me. My imagination can't invent a "voice" out of thin air - it does require an actual sound ("external stimuli") – a low rumble of a clothes dryer, static from a transistor radio, evening crickets, a dog's distant bark. Like finding images in fluffy clouds, "seeing" something in something else, I can "hear" words inside other noises. When a certain thought won't go away, I might recognize it in a magazine headline or TV commercial or hear it in a stranger's conversation. It becomes affirmation that my obsession "means something" beyond just my imagination. Affirmation that something in the world is shifting, the external and internal blending together because I've anticipated a real event that is suddenly coming true. New Age Synchronicities are not so new to everybody. And not so appealing. "I've been feeling a lot better" I tell Dr. S on Thursday. Then out of nowhere, 24 hours later at home - it's night, and warm, too warm. So my fan is turned on high speed, the blades whir, but unevenly… there's a syncopation, a two syllable count. "wir..uh…wir…uh…" faster as I focus to listen. Wir-ruh, wi-ruh, wi-duh, wee-duh…window, window, window. And sudden panic. I've thought before about suiciding from a window. From one or another, wouldn't matter which. No, not to go there, try not to, anyway. Defenestrate means to jump from a window, and the dictionary was nearby... With these thoughts I'm terrified and enthralled. "Window" is its voice; the fan lives in perpetual motion. The thought of unplugging it feels murderous. "Better jump before ya kill." I think it, not hear it. I know it's my internal voice. I guess. Or maybe I tell myself I'm telling myself...maybe the words are that warning. It could finally be time to find out what things really mean. Definitions royal? Or plant the soil, and know it's all just speeches and cream. The fan is no longer an object. I forget it has blades that cut through air. Because words are the only real cutters. It all starts that way, just a toss of the stone and you jump on the One. Anybody can pick up from One! And by the time ya get to Ten, kids get bored and they laugh or they leave. Windowwindowwindow.... But it's not now. Widow. A widow. That's what he'd be – if I had a husband, if I ever wanted one – and I don't. Why do people want things I don't want? And why do they watch me so much? Why do they keep eyes on me if I won't be like them? I'm not hurting anybody. I never would, and the killer is I don't even hurt myself. But he'd be a widow, no widower, isn't that the word? More fear when I can't remember the right word! I just don't want anyone to live with me, don't want anyone to touch me every day and that makes me strange. Sick. My mind jumps to the wrong word first, it isn't right. Just jump, you stupid child. My thought? Who can tell?

Window.

And I'm there.

Every word suddenly links to some cliché. Every phrase brings its sound-alike or a bad pun. The frantically-paced rambling must sound mad, disconnected, but it is actually an effort at ultimate connection. A word association game with survival to the winner. Back and forth in time, thoughts go – and with that, I think of a watch. "Watch" leads my mind to "Don't Look Now" an old movie with Julie Christie; it was scary, scared me into a state... Julie Christie sounds like Christ – and then a return to the word "time" joins in and it's too late, it suddenly means The Second Coming – then "come" leads to orgasm. It's now too hot, way way too dark. Too dangerous. Thoughts of children's nursery rhymes, anything before the age of sex. Let thinking be pure, be safe.... Let every thought bring more than spring rain, and see, seeing sea shells really is a trap. I'd never scare a mouse, I'd

27

just let them crawl into pickled peppers, but words come easy and talk is cheap, thought the little canary (and would've said so if he could talk). Birds know two. They're the best. And not because some ABC motherfucker says "Father Knows…" and who doesn't hate the 1950's?! I remember Betty pretty well, and Bud I guess, but she was never a favorite of mine. Oh, yeah, if not mine, then whose? In King Solomon's world that old movie about his Mines, but it had such a big spider that got on Deborah Kerr's skirt. A hand print touching her thigh. No not her leg, just her canvas skirt… but the goddamn insect was just too big, although it was all those movie stars' huge tits that made them call their studio MGM. Could anyone imagine how much I want to tell these thoughts? Sometimes I wish another person could think alongside me for just five minutes. They wouldn't have to risk anything, I'd let them be a passive passenger, no driving required… to be able to find a way to finally tell it. "Just try to talk" Strauss said to me. "You can tell me whatever you're feeling…" No. I CAN'T. You have no fucking clue how fast my mind can run, too fast to ever try to say. "They're only thoughts. That's all." Then you do not understand! "Stay with me a minute – yes, they're fast. They have to be – to keep you BUSY – busy enough that you don't have to be aware of how you feel…" I can't hear this. Can't hear you right now. Please remember what you're saying, and try me again when I'm a little clearer. It's different, what you're saying. But I can't hear. And tonight, you're not even with me. You're probably talking to someone else in your golden lit room, a patient with a late evening appointment. Someone who rates. I sit alone, and want to be alone. I just don't want to be me.

Cutting a wrist? Would help would would would woodlewoood wood. Until I scratch my forearm hard and deep, but still not deep enough to cut. I'm alive. Awake. I am awake, no dream. The thin piece of metal from a pen in my hand sharp edge digs to my arm, of my arm, at it. Wrong prepositions can't make plasma appear. Deeper and blood, but no violence, no one was mad. I sit on the floor, safe from heights. I crawl like a little kid, in a silly way. I crawl to the phone and act silly. No laughing. It's gonna be okay. "Dr. Strauss, this is Janine. If you can, if you have a chance, could ya call me? I was thinking it's not an emergency…" But I don't explain. In fact, I never even dial the phone. I say the words only in my head. No mention of a cut to feel real. Thought about it, didn't even tilt the blade. No big deal. So no need to say it out loud. No windows. Don't want anyone to think I'm crazy.

In the morning I carry the fan to the street. It stands next to garbage cans for 26 hours. I know it's there. When will they come? They should have taken it already. At 4 a.m. the next day, my savior truck arrives and loads it in. They have literally given back my life, and I consider pulling the shades up and my nightgown as well. Showing them some tits for their trouble. I want to press my breasts against the cold glass, and finally laugh at the thought of touching a window. They look up. I realize they couldn't hear what I was thinking. I do realize that. Then I hear a screech as the compactor crushes the fan. What have I done? "Better jump before ya kill..." I remember. In a flood, I remember. The next two hours I lie in an empty bathtub, cold and uncomfortable enough to keep me awake. No matter what, I cannot let myself sleep. Later at work when I'm exhausted, and know I've said too much, one of the secretaries tries empathy. "It's *terrible* when ya can't get to sleep," she says. "I really understand..."

For the rest of the afternoon, I laugh to myself off and on, remembering what she said.

They have no idea, the idiots at work.

I came back from the bathroom and not one of them has a clue.

"So where does this doctor think your panic comes from?" Casey asks a few weeks later.

"Who knows?" Laughing at the unfunny as only I can. "He keeps talking about strong feelings trying to break through...I've read about that before. But it's not me. I've had this too long."

"Does it seem like he'll be able to help you?"

"Yeah, I like him. Very nice, and I think he's helping already. Today, it came over me just cause of PMS. That's what set it off..." Reassure her. Soothe her. It's okay.

"You're drinking orange juice. I've seen you do that before when you get anxious...maybe it's a form of hypoglycemia. Ever notice if you feel better or worse after eating certain food?" For the next couple of hours we explore that idea together. There does seem to be a pattern. When I eat too much sugar with no protein,

29

I'm *much* more likely to feel bad. We try to reconstruct past anxiety attacks and trace the villains to a bad meal combo. In her invaluable overkill style, my dear friend makes a calendar grid on her computer with times of day, space to write menus, and a few lines for descriptions of how I felt afterwards. She is kind, so determined to help. I promise to use the log religiously and she suggests I share it Strauss, telling him what I've noticed. Oh, yeah, that'll go over big. "Wouldn't it be something?" she grins, "if this turns out to be the missing piece?" I smile back, feeling considerably better. Calves liver, anyone?

"Well, *sure* ya felt better!" he slams Casey's theory into dust. "The two of you working together, trying to solve your problem... must've felt a lot like you and your grandmother..." He's jealous. Ten years of education, medical school, internship. How could Casey and I figure out this puzzle when we're mere lay people? "Look, there might be *something* to your diet...too much sugar can make anybody edgy, and too much caffeine. But I want you to see what else you were getting out of that time with Casey, besides nutrition advice." He smiles. It's not his fault. Nobody can know everything.

"Yeah, I see what you're saying," I concede. "But I still want to keep this log..."

"Okay" he says. Please don't be mad.

Strauss just shakes his head a little sadly when I confess that I already know what he wants me to say. But truth is, I'm right, and it seems I'm getting to know him better and faster than he's understanding *me*. Patterns. Re-woven, re-lived over and fucking over.

"You're really tired today," I say, his eyes heavy as I enter the room. He only laughs.

"Quite the opposite" he lies. "Maybe *you* are. Hmm? Was that describing how you're feeling?" Interesting that I'm not the only one who hides.

"...The only thing I've asked of you is to just say whatever comes to your mind..." Free association. Nothing in life is free.

You claim you want to help me not keep looking at everything *one* way – to be able to *revise* how I've thought for so long. My god, look how many times I've *already* revised myself, the world... It's the *problem*, not the answer. We've heading the wrong way into a tunnel.

I have a hundred voices and can look from a thousand different angles. The people I care about...I can see them as evil, I can see them as saints. Life is precious, life is shit. I can picture myself a wealthy movie star, beloved, bedazzled, begrudged, despised. And just as easily, I could be one never seen at all – a homeless crazy who sleeps in the streets and hollers at strangers who won't look in her eyes. I am everything. I am nothing. I'm the Wisest. I am deaf, dumb and blind.

I'm a seagull. No, an actress. That's how we know poor Nina's mad. Self-image loose in the atmosphere. *Who am I?* People laugh as if it's a silly question, when in fact, it is a question of life and death because I live every day in terror of the answer. No, not to find out I'm nobody – that would be almost a relief. The unthinkable truth is that I am everyone.

I am the world itself, my thoughts are the wind in the trees, my anger is the snowstorm, my fears are the fires.

My Self. All there is, ever was, or ever will be. Amen. But there are no prayers in hell.

None of this is in Strauss's ears. He is a different kind of man. It would make no sense to him. He'd only ask why I don't want to have more friends.

Cleo still is not feeling well. The woman who is never sick. Not feeling well. But there's no one I want to tell.

Madness is time gone haywire. Yesterday could be twenty years ago.

He laughs, a man with a round face and hardly any hair. I'm nearly fifteen and for the past several months, my life has been changing. He's everywhere lately. That face, big open mouth just laughing. It's not that I *see* things, but I sort of spy him. Like "Where's Waldo?" there are always faces hiding in a variety of daily sights. His eyes are also round with crinkles in their corners. Not that he looks happy exactly. No, that couldn't be said. He's laughing only to *seem* jovial, and it's a social grease job gone a bit too far. There's this pile of clothes in my bedroom, always. Since I was born or before I suppose. Clothes folded neatly way down at the bottom of the stack, but higher up, more things, and then more, have been tossed without a thought or excuse. Probably wrinkled by now, piled high by now, a couple of towels, then one of my old skirts...and that's where it is... there in one of my blouses - his face. I've seen it for a few months now, but managed to resist looking too close. My specialty. Periphery. Glimmer. "Hints of..." can't hurt anyone. From such distance, the poor guy seems harmless. Just watching is all. It's okay in a way that I have such a remarkable imagination. And now, finally...it seems I'm pretending decent things. Only a happy man. This may be what it is to grow up, and if so, oh, not so bad. Monsters aren't real, ghosts aren't real. And, no longer a child, I smile and shake my head. What if Cleo's been right? Those made-up things are told to scare kids, not real, just stories....I'll be 15 so soon, and with that day, the sun comes up a different color. It's possible.

"Cleo! When you get a chance, can you come?!"

"On my way!"

I want to tell her that I'm doing so much better. More than that, she needs to know the worst is finally over. Opening the bedroom door, she balances a glass jar filled with iced tea, always knowing what I want. Her dress is damp ("I was just rinsing out some old towels..."). But it's not water, it's sweat.

"I wish you didn't have to work in this heat." I stroke her hand, cool and smooth because we always know what the other of us wants.

"Oh I don't mind," she takes my fingers and kisses them. "I just keep drinking good cold ice water. You look like you're feeling better!" I glance back to the face in the clothes. It looks smaller when she's in the room. I talk about feeling hopeful again, looking forward to my birthday now. As always she hangs on every word. And I hang onto her, to her hands, to her thoughts, unsure who is saying what and who's listening. To make a cake or buy one? What presents do I think of? A remarkable afternoon of normal pleasures.

When my mother gets home from work at four, Cleo tells her that I'm feeling well now, so much stronger and we're planning a strawberry shortcake for next week. My mother's timid knock on the bedroom door, so unpredictable that timidity. Whether to rush or slink. Hard decisions for any predator lacking Darwinian advantage. So cautious around me, her only child, flesh and blood

32

and all of that. I understand. I don't feel at home in *her* room either. We have always been each others' eggshells. But I'm feeling too good to hate her right then. I even smile while looking right into her eyes. It may have been the last time I ever did.

Then to Cleo "before you start supper, I want to take a bath..." That means I need her in there with me, to sit nearby and talk. Or listen. To be. To let me ramble in the way that protects me. Naked and cold, always too cold in the tub, but hot water makes me feel strange. I'll just talk and keep talking and the joyous normal plans we make will keep everyone warm. I walk to the pile of clothes and beneath Mr. Laughter, I reach for the softest red towel. Images shift, new folds reveal more. He is not only a face, I can see that now. I see his hands. The room moves. And my eyes dart side to side. I watch it happen, feel me happen. Watching and being, seeing and feeling, it's too much. Can't breathe. A wild heat from head to toe, like my life itself is leaving me. Rush, a rush, a brush and flushed face but I never turn colors, can't breathe! More heat. It touches, and it's like a giant swarm of flapping insects racing down me, up me, around me, inside me. Like a thick scalding liquid. "I'm drowning!! CLEO!"

Her legs don't seem to be moving right, and then I hear running, and the sound of that, her age, her feet, backwards, wrong, scuffing that could be leading the other way! "Cleo!"

"Oh, honey, honey!" Her arms around me. I stare at the floor to find a spot, FIND YOUR POINT, GIRL, try to focus, fists clenched, fingernails dig in my hand – I can't feel!

"I can't feel! I can't...breathe..." Go slow, just slow. Slow down. Show it down...a final final show down of them all.

"What is it?!" Mary Jane at the door.

"She's okay," frantic Cleo. "She stood up too fast..." If I stare at the floor – my toes, toenails look right. It's there, solid, the floor...not a square but more rounded across the top...my foot not the floor.

"Is a rectangle bigger than a square?" I beg.

"I don't know, honey..." Cleo hugs and holds and strokes and I feel. "I don't know. It's all right..." She hands me some water and I hold it against my face. Sudden cold, flashes of cold can help...try to remember, remember what helps...

"This is it!" I gasp. "My hands can't feel. I can't feel my hands!" She takes them again and holds tighter. Mary Jane talks, but its far away. Just too close in the biggest scheme of things. "Please" I beg Cleo. "Nobody else, right now. Please ask her to go back ..." Don't let her start, can't take her starting, Cleo's apron/my face/on her lap, the damp cloth, smells of vegetables and Tide. The taste/odor of onions and raw potatoes will stay a lifelong perfume. Whatever sounds of her, tastes of her is safe. And that alone. Any other berry must not be eaten.

"I saw something..." I try. And pull away. I honest to god really do sometimes try. "No, its okay, don't hold me..."

"Was it outside? Out the window?" I don't shake my head or bother with "no." I will not tell her, can't bear to hear myself say it. It didn't happen. I was thinking is all...Cleo's words are muffled now, and can tell my self is sliding as the light from the window gets brighter. Too bright. And too many people can tell. "Can you catch your breath now?" That I do *not* know. Nor how long I'll live. If I'm right, and the time is over...

"Was whatever you saw...was it something out there?"

"Please, don't say it, okay? Please please please please..."

"Okay, okay.." She is scared and god damn us all to hell, *that* I can feel. Please no. *I'm all right...* "Of course you are..."

"Just promise never say anything about this ever..." Past her nodding head, I glance back at the clothes. A laughing man's face, and he's looking ahead. A head. He gestures with arms he doesn't see, and at the end of each arm at the wrist, sliced clean, blood pours. Both of his hands have been hacked off and now lay beneath him, one hidden in another fold of fabric, one lying still numb and frozen.

He hasn't seen, yet.

He does not know.

And for the last time, before he looks down, for one last instant, still without having to know, he laughs.

Over the next five years, I think about it every day and "see" the man in a thousand forms. A foolhardy bellower and his unseen severed limbs. Sometimes no feet. Or only missing fingers. In patterns, in pictures, in rugs, on signs. I see it. And say nothing.

Nor do I choose to tell that since that day, the world has belonged to another dimension. When I wake up, everything around me is the same as when I slept. A Dali painting, the heart of a deep REM sleep. No shadow looks like that in waking life, no angle, no depth...people are cardboard, outlined in ink...and I eat and I smile and I talk without knowing if I'm awake. And I wait for anything. In dreams, where anything can happen.

Oh, we were supposed to have a different ending, Cleo. I was going to bring you up here to live with me, after I got better, after Casey became a huge star...they would've died first, your children, I'm sorry but they would (in the way I planned things out) and you and me and lots of money, we'd have all the time in the world.

"My grandmother died last night..." What a way to start a session.

"Oh, I am *so sorry*..." Everyone is. I'm surrounded by pure compassion today, and even more precious, by distance. They're letting me be anyway I need. I knew she was dying, no need to say so now...well, I knew it for forty years. But today, the day where everyone is being dear, the sun came up and I went to work. This, the first evening she is not in the world, and I am still alive, still as sane (well as I ever was). Strauss keeps glancing for my grief, and I'm open, babe. Where should we look? Cause the hell of it all is I feel okay, and I should cry but I've cried so much for this event. And now after it all, she's merely dead. No one judges even that, they nod and say it's hard...I'm forgiven everything and given that, well, it's clear I'm the evil prick I always thought. In many ways, this has been the easiest day of my life.

Like everything, the anti-climax of the worst loss I will ever know. Shells of people can make a nice seating arrangement if ya don't focus on the fact that no one's breathing. Let's dress the windows and play the game. Everyone cares. They do.

It's just that nobody gives a shit.

Thursday 6 p.m.

It really doesn't bother me, but I do find it *interesting* he's always late. I would've never figured this conventional doctor for

35

a rule breaker. According to my home library, the "therapeutic frame" should stay consistent – time and place of sessions, the fee, procedures, the rules. Prompt. Dependable. In most ways, he is orthodox – mature, warm but formal. Kinda reserved. Appropriate for a classically-trained analyst. Freudian impulses, slips of the tongue, manifest dream content are peppered in his conversation. "*Everyone* has conflicts," he's said more than twice. Apparently so, since "sorry-to-keep-ya-waiting" is his version of hello. I imagine that occasionally the patient before me has had a small crisis, but the man is late even when there's absolutely nobody in there with him. "It's no big deal" I reassure. "Once in a while it matters, only because I can't always be late getting back to work…" He seems to understand and says he'll try to make it a point to be more punctual (which sounds to me like "more pregnant"). It's okay. Everybody needs illusions. At this point, I could be left out there for half an hour, and wouldn't mention it, because I'm figuring out the structure to these sessions. He takes whatever I say in the first few minutes as the subject my unconscious mind has chosen for Theme of the Day. Yeah, as if. As if I could ever let my fucking unconscious make any decisions. The poor guy has no idea that I literally rehearse my comments. I decide what symptoms to talk about, and exactly how much to divulge and when. I have to. I'd tell you so, if I thought you could hear. It's not because I'm controlling or manipulative or because I don't trust you. But the soft milky paste that does such a flimsy job holding my mind together can't take any surprises. That much I have told you. I'm taking care of myself for both of us, keeping me from going psychotic under your care. I know who I am and I know what I'm doing. Granted, I'm not better. I'm also not *worse*.

Lower your standards, White Rabbit. Every day, I forgive *you* your tardiness.

Monday 6 p.m. Over a year now.

Of Mondays.

And nothing is different. All my life I suppose I've harbored the greatest fantasy of all – that with the right doctor, the right medication, it could be fixed. I know better, knew it all along. But I was a pathetic child lost in the store who'll fly into any mother's arms.

36

Within several months, Otis is dead. And then Mary Jane. Of course. Most people can't survive once their Life Support is disconnected. They're gone. All of them. I should feel...something.

On and on I go about Otis and his threats – gone now, no one killed after all. He was never mean to us, but the things he said he wanted to do to other people. Vengeance. Tortures. Seared into my soul.

"But it's not about how frightening something *was* – we can't do anything to change that." I listen, and some of it makes sense.

"Don't you think it explains a lot though? Of why I'm so afraid all the time, why I freak out..."

"Sure, it can explain part of it. But the bigger part, and this is the part we can work on, is how you've put things together in your mind. We can't change the past, but hopefully, we can revise how you react to it."

A childhood of fear. It's almost like Post-traumatic stress – of course I'm an anxious wreck. For a year, Dr. Strauss has reassured that I won't go crazy and not be able to get back to reality. I'll make it, and I even tell Casey that I'm feeling stronger. I reassure her because no one would want to have a friend in a mental home. I understand. Hey, I understand.

Then from nowhere, four days where I couldn't get to work. I was one block from home when the world changed. Buildings are made of red brick and that *is* the color, red, it is... But I saw something today, the side of one store...I saw a color that has never been seen. Was not red, was not brown...not a special shade, but an entirely new color. And they say that is impossible. The mind cannot invent such a thing, can only modify, not truly create form from nothing. Yet I did. I witnessed something that's never been seen before or since. And it all started happening. I could literally feel it. My hands were paper. The flesh was stale, no blood had ever flowed and I knew if I shook them, they would flutter like wings of tissue. No breath. Of course I was breathing, I was standing, I was living...but if my hands were not real, then where would oxygen go? I'd freeze when it reached my wrists. My hands belonged to someone else. I recognized them, I understood reality, but something was very wrong, something so different. I can never explain it right, words aren't the right words... but my breathing didn't sound like mine either. Aware of a self that isn't me, but of me, in me and in a world within a world like nested Russian dolls, a smaller one inside another and then one more, always more, inside that one. Infinity. Replicated realities, alternate views of a world in a world that eventually cancel themselves out, and from limitless numbers comes zero. Nothing was left and when we finally understood everything, had learned it all, at that instant, we were left in dark silence as if we'd never been born. For god's sake, you idiot girl, you're dreaming. Do you remember getting up this morning, think back...you're still lying in bed safe with flesh hands. The human mind cannot invent a color. Hundreds of dreams where I know I am dreaming, frantic pleas to awaken, terror of a victim waiting to be destroyed by anything imagination can conjure. Even a color never seen? In a nightmare, I know what to do, a technique used hundreds of times, I fly from a height, to crash on the ground...hands right in front of me, watching the earth spin closer, hands touch...and then...touch and fade. And sleep is murdered. But if by chance, I was wrong, if by chance I was not dreaming...well, then what a very irreparable error, wouldn't ya say? I've been so positive I was awake - and been dead wrong. If I wrongly believe I'm dreaming, I'll die in my effort to survive.

"Why would you need to destroy yourself to wake up?" Yeah, well, live every day not knowing if you're real and then get back to me.

All the buildings in the street have become two-dimensional. They're flats from an old movie set, cardboard images that look like actual buildings from one angle, but turn a head and they become drawings. Smoke and mirrors. Think it's funny, bastard? People keep walking, no one else sees. Of course they don't see it. No one is alive anyway. I made up the whole show— every person, every sound, every light that won't change, every street I can't cross. It's all some dream I dreamed before I died.

"What do you think brought it on?" I don't *know*. Please hear me. I do not know. "That's why I keep saying it's chemical. Something in my brain just clicks..."

"It would help if we try to examine what you were thinking when it started…" Yes. I understand that. I don't *know*. "If ya can't remember, tell me whatever you're thinking of right now…"

"Just the fact that it'll never stop."

"That what won't stop?" No hidden meaning there, Sigmund. I only mean my madness. My hell.

"What are ya thinking now?" Leave me alone.

That night I imagine Jack insisting that Connor try to talk. Pushing her. Trying to help. Something's not right. Their words in my head are too much like our words in that room. I will borrow from movies, take lines from a script, but I will be damned (and so will you) if I ever let some real person's words slide into my mind.

Connor is my ultimate secret, the one kept even from Cleo. A wild girl, angry and bitter and underneath, yeah, probably not so bad, but on the surface, that dangerous ground where people meet… she is nothing but pure hell. And in this fantasy character and her hostile interactions with the world, I find my sex. In her battles with teachers, with guardians at the orphanage where she was raised, in everyone's struggle with her hatred…I find pleasure. It is not something to share or brag about. It is my private sanctum of hidden night, and guarantees that no one else, no one real could ever do it as well. I know me, my buttons, the heat of my mind. The schmucks at Lara's paid for what I can do alone.

Lately, when Strauss and I debate back and forth, I find it useful as fodder for those thoughts. Instead of some teacher, there's now a doctor with Connor. He's still part of the Establishment of course, all that crap that speaks to the masses…but he's not the jerk some of the other characters were. He's not the horrible man who usually appears in these thoughts. Still, she's a bit much for him, she is, as he tries techniques and rattles his brain, and she only rattles his cage. The entrapment he doesn't see.

Thursday 7 p.m.

"Any plans for the holidays?" he asks.

"Christmas is Casey's day – the whole season, actually. So, yes...with her. Whatever she wants." Then I catch it. "Not in some *sacrificing* way" I laugh. "But it's important to her, so I gladly play."

"It's not important to you?" Yes, should've seen it coming.

"In a way. But I'm not much of a holiday person."

Over the years, Casey's worked to change that. We give tons of gifts, and not especially costly ones. Handmade ornaments take the most time, and are the most rewarding. We make them to commemorate some event from the year, something we shared...most are hilarious, some very touching. The Christmas tree becomes a photo album of memories...

"Sometimes we can be "Mom" to each other in *good* ways, I guess," I say, looking for a little approval. "Cleo used to buy me lots of stuffed animals, I loved them, didn't like dolls. Then Casey started it, and I've got this wonderful teddy bear collection that rivals FAO Schwartz. A few years back somebody came out with a line of "famous bears." Queen Eliza-bear, the Van DerBear Family, ...all dressed in appropriate costumes. Well, that Christmas I got Janine Bear-ker, dressed exactly like me – literally, cause Casey had stolen some of my old knock-arounds and cut and sewn a little outfit..."

He smiles. "Special attention, like Cleo."

Yeah. Well, I play, too. When Casey was growing up, every Easter her younger brothers and sisters always got up before her, hunted down her chocolate rabbit and bit the ears off before she woke up. The family thought it was funny, cute...it became a family story... But to her, it was a painful metaphor. No matter how much she complained and begged them, nobody could get them to stop. So she never got a single rabbit with ears intact. The first Easter after we met I gave her a huge basket filled with colored grass and decorated with ribbons. With nothing inside except 25 tied-up little plastic baggies – each contained a set of chocolate rabbit ears..."

"Enormously clever," he grins. "Now on the *analytic* front...you were trying to *undo* her bad memories.."

"Yeah. Sure."

"Slippery turf." Yeah. Sure. But there's nothing we treasure more than the things we never got.

And the dreadful morning that brings only work. I suppose I could feel pleased with my new official job. The temp position has suddenly turned permanent, an offer, a yes...and done. I must admit I'm thrilled about it being in one of the classiest office buildings in New York. Midtown, right in the heart of the most wonderful city in the world. Not bad for a chick who used to be that word we don't use.

The ever-supportive Casey has gone shopping with me, picked out the "right" silk blouses, wool suits, and classic shoes. When I walk through the mahogany doors, smile at our receptionist, and stroll down a burgundy-carpeted hallway, I can't believe it's even me. Like other people. Nice people. Different. From who I really am.

"So ya *like* the new firm." A smiling doctor, pleased when his patient does well. And that too, is nice. What I can't say, of course, is that we are acting proud because I'm working as a fucking secretary! If I hadn't been crazy, I might have been a college teacher, or a scientist. I would have lived a life with people as brilliant as the voices I read in books. I could have been a person whom others admired, not patronized. My thoughts could have challenged, not soothed them, not flattered and stroked them into coming. If I hadn't been crazy, I might not have become a whore.

"They all like me there. I'm doing a decent job of fitting in..."

"...or you're pretending to be a certain way and *getting* them to like you?"

"Well said. Mostly I'm scared of what will happen if I get panicky..." Then he launches into wondering why I anticipate such a thing. What might make me anxious there? Why would I need to do that to myself? Poor thing, he was almost hopeful I'd be leaving soon. "Anyway, it feels weird to dress up every day, you know, to look nice. At Lara's I dressed like a slob..." He never probes into what went on there. I acted out sexual fantasies, boy. How can that not be on your mind every time I walk into this room?

After the session, I walk into a drug store to fill the even-more-important-than-ever valium script and catch a glimpse of myself on a security camera. Maybe I've been overestimating this new façade. It's still me, still my visibly uncomfortable, postured look. When I hand over the prescription, they must think "sure, figured it'd be a tranquilizer..." Some people just can't look natural in their own skin. The good news is that I clearly don't look my age. Heredity promises that in my family one can keep looking young way past the time insanity sets in. Soft skin, delicate features, great bones, and oh, yeah, that pesky psychosis.

"Mama, come look at this picture!" Mary Jane's shrill voice down the hall. "Janine looks just like her!" Cleo scurried into the room, so eager when the yelling was cheerful. "It's Scarlett! Janine looks exactly like Vivian Leigh!" First of all, I really didn't. Secondly, I was eight. But to Mommy, the most important question about anyone was "well, who do they look like?" Mary Jane's bedroom was covered in movie star photos, carefully torn from magazines, and scotch taped directly to the walls. Plastic curtains hung over windows, a lamp from Woolworth's sat in the center of a dresser littered with dusty costume jewelry, and overseeing the whole world gazed Jean Harlow, Lana Turner, Kim Novak. They were like goddesses at Delphi blessing her hovel, smiling and posing just for Mary Jane. We were all damn good at looking past the dirt, around the clutter, and focusing only on what we chose to see. "Mama, you looked like Vivian Leigh when you were younger too!"

"Oh, no, I think Janine looks more like her!" Cleo stepping aside in the way that made us adore her. "I look more like Jane Wyman."

"That's right, that's right..." Cleo had also been compared to Patricia Neal in the new movie with Paul Newman. "We need to go see that again. She looks more like you than ever!"

Otis was David Janssen from *The Fugitive* so we couldn't miss an episode. Mary Jane had a longer list than the rest of us, since her own personal style changed like weather. Betty Grable, when she was younger, Lana Turner, Ann Southern. In her darker hair phase, she could see "a little Rita Hayworth, just around the mouth..." As middle age crept up and her body deferred to years of medications she starting admitting Simone Signoret and at her fattest, Shelley Winters. The honesty and relative accuracy of her self-image was such a funny piece of reality. Why not just believe you looked like whoever you *wanted*? If you're gonna live your whole fucking life in a fantasy world, why defer to things like *weight*? "I always call 'em like I see 'em..." she prided herself. "Once I really had "*It*" but now I don't... and I know it...." And when Cleo tried to reassure that her figure was as beautiful as ever, she only shrugged her shoulders and said "Mama, you have delusions." Even madness has ground rules.

A bad day at work, leaving early. Beginning of the end.

The madness is in my genes, but you don't seem to believe me anymore. I can't take one more accusation that I do this to myself!

"I'm not sure you're hearing me on this," offers Dr. Energy Bunny... on and on and on. "When I point out that you bring on those feelings, I'm not casting blame, not at all. But if you can see the part you play in it, you can stop it from happening..."

"Why would you think I would possibly bring such a thing on myself?"

"It's a defense – designed by *you* – unconsciously – to protect against something..." I nod. It's not crap, I've read things like this. He's trying. More is said. Clock hands move. I nod again. I endure. It's in my genes.

"You tell me so much about how your mother acted. It's made a huge impression on you, her schizophrenia. I think you tried very hard to understand her..." No. I had no interest in her whatsoever. "That's not true, it's not even possible. All little children are fascinated by their mothers..." I was not like other children.

"Mama! Look at the little girl who's playing Gregory Peck's daughter!!" The other second graders didn't get to see *To Kill A Mockingbird*. It seems their parents doubted that rape, Southern racism and hour-long courtroom scenes were good entertainment for seven-year olds. But I was destined to see it because I was a dead-ringer for Scout. Mary Jane took the day off from work. Actually, that sounds too autonomous – what she actually did was get so excited about the prospect of seeing it that she had an anxiety attack in her morning bath so Cleo called the restaurant saying her poor daughter had an upset stomach and couldn't come in, leaving Mary Jane with newfound freedom to spend the day with Gregory Peck.

"I shouldn't have let her go to that show alone..." Cleo self-tortured later that night. Having sat through the movie two and a half times, she was more able than ever to repeat the movie word for word.

"Do you understand, Mama?!" Way too loud, way too excited. "It was his daughter! Gregory Peck's! The one who looks just like Janine!" Cleo understood that my biological father had looked a lot like Mr. Peck, and although he meant nothing to her daughter, he was, granted, the guy with the sperm. ("Is he *always* here?" Mary Jane asked once, as if his genes in my face meant an intruder was constantly watching).

For the next 72 hours, no one really slept. I dozed off periodically, but woke up to her ramblings about Addicus Finch and his little girl and the summer that changed everyone's lives. Otis insisted the movies can drive a person crazy, but Cleo insisted it sounded like an excellent picture, thanking Mary Jane for her reports, and desperately looking for any signs of sleepiness. By the weekend, she was tired, and Saturday night brought safety. We lay in bed, all of us, for once on a shared timetable, connected through psychotic exhaustion. In my own mind, I played scenes from the movie I hadn't even seen yet. Cleo and I went together the following week, and it was kinda amazing how much I resembled that kid. "Her bangs are way over her eyebrows just like yours!" It became our summer movie, and I became Scout.

A few years later, my look-alike evolved into Natalie Wood ("not the way she was in *West Side Story*" – which yes, I'd also seen at age 6 – "but how she looks in this new one, *Inside Daisy Clover...*") Ms. Clover was sporting my signature overgrown bangs. I vowed to let mine grow in a useless effort to avoid the *Who Am I?* game, and more importantly, to avoid her gaze. Within a few months, my forehead was clear and I joyously parted my hair low on one side. It seemed such a good idea until some ominous events began rearing their bangless heads.

Our trouble started with *Coming Attractions* for the new picture *This Property Is Condemned* starring Robert Redford and Natalie Wood ("the *exact* same twosome from *Daisy Clover*!!") Nothing uncanny about two actors being paired up again when they have good chemistry. Even Nut Job had to see that. But meaningful coincidences were only beginning. It seems that *Property* opened with a scene on an abandoned train track where an adolescent girl was playing dress-up in clothes that once belonged to her sister (our Natalie). The girl then proceeded to tell her (now dead) sister's tragic story in flashbacks. The girl was "Scout." That once darling kid from *Mockingbird* had not grown up to be quite as cute. Boyish, gawky, almost homely, but the little bitch still had those damn long bangs. "And you don't!" Mary Jane squealed and people steered clear of us as we left the theatre. "She's not like you anymore, sweet thing! Oh, what happened to her? She's not even pretty now. You knew! You knew!"

It gets worse. Natalie Wood had made some changes of her own. She'd begun parting her hair low on one side.

Trying to lay it all out with mere logic is impossible, but filtered through Mary Jane's unshakeable passion, the synchronicity spoke volumes. "You started wearing your hair like that last year! You knew!!!"

All I knew was that I'd had it. In a moment of anger, rage probably, but not of craziness, not at all, I raced into the house, grabbed a pair of scissors and hacked off my hair. I was not anxious or out of it, I was not dreaming or delusional. I was fed up. First to the shoulders, then below the ears, up and up, one side and the other, shorter and madder and madder and shorter. In making my statement, I sort of forgot that my locks are kinda think and not the easiest hair in the world to work with. Such a super-short cut was not a well though-out cosmetic choice, but fuck us all, it was done. Kind of "pixie," I practiced. My face is pretty enough, small features. It's not bad. It's short all right. It's done. By nightfall I was almost pleased with it. Cleo said it was "very different" and Otis added that it would dry very fast now. All in all it wasn't a big deal – at least for a week.

The following Saturday brought a morning paper that changed our lives. A few months earlier, Mia Farrow, one of our beloved favorites of television's *Peyton Place*, had surprised Hollywood by starting to date Frank Sinatra. Barely twenty years old. Fifty-one years old. Innocent maiden. Rat Pack kingpin. Virgin princess, powerful rogue…(See *Mary Jane* for full psychological profiles). Naturally it had been a House Topic lately, and then that morning paper. It seemed that our gentle little

45

Mia had gotten pissed at ol' Blue Eyes. The other night they'd had a fight, the two stars had, over another woman, who knows/who cares, but they had a bad fight, and afterwards, Mia had for whatever reason, chopped off her waist-length blond hair leaving only about three inches of golden fuzz on top of her head. It didn't look too bad though. Underneath the picture on the front page was a caption that said she now looked like a pixie. There just wasn't enough Thorazine in the world.

"Can you see why I need a lot of privacy now?" I chuckle. "I've already had way too much companionship." Sometimes the man doesn't feel like laughing.

"What about other people in your life – *besides* Casey? Seems you put all your eggs in that one basket..." He is such a nice guy, but hardly quotable.

"I have other friends."

"You rarely mention them. They don't seem very important to you."

"But that's not part of all this." Whose treatment are we doing? "*People* are not the problem. If I wanted more friends in my life, I could have them tomorrow."

"Got it all figured out." I see the disapproval loud and clear. Luckily I just don't care.

"I've *had* love - with my grandmother, with Casey ... we can talk like this if you want to, but..." But the hour's half gone. Another session bites the dust.

"It's just that relationships are pretty important to most people..." I hope you can see my face. "But don't do it for *me*. As always, what we talk about is up to you." Good.

"Thanks. Anyway, people... just take too much energy." Even this conversation does.

He takes a sip of coffee. "How come?" Visible panty-line. Your fly is open. Excuse me, doctor, but in a blatant and rather repulsive way, your technique is showing.

"Please don't."

"I don't understand. What is it you think I did?" Uh, huh...don't do *that* either.

"Never mind. It's okay..." is all I say. Why can't anyone be seamless? You honestly think I don't see the transparency of your effort at being casual? That off-handed "how come?" said with coffee but without vigor, without valence, without a hint of passion. You think by down-playing your interest in my answer, you can trick me into some benign little walk down the lane? That must work with some people, and that is astounding to me. A photographer took some pictures when I was seventeen. He said I could be a model and we took some shots. After about twenty minutes, he suggested oh, so casually, that I might want to unbutton my blouse a little, and even another button if I wanted, in-fact-I-could-slip-it-off-one-shoulder-no-big-deal-just-a-thought. I laughed and told him he was barking up the wrong virgin, got my stuff and left. Actually what I said was that I wasn't feeling well and could I come back next week instead, and I smiled when I said it and I showed some tit (off-handedly, accidentally) so he wouldn't get mad and try to kill me. I let him see enough to think I was interested, to keep him hoping so he wouldn't hurt me right away, would want me to come back again...and not come in for the kill too fast. Sometimes that's all you can ask for. I kissed him on the cheek as I left, promising next Saturday at noon. I led him on to save my life. Well, sometimes you have to. People take so much energy.

"So what was it you thought I did just now?" He won't let it go. Maybe what I thought you did is what you were doing. How's that for mental health?

"When you ask it like that, you're implying I was delusional." I do smile when I say it.

"Oh, boy, is that what you heard in my question?" I give up. What would you like to hear?

"Maybe I felt pressured." I offer. "I guess that must be it." Here, let me slide myself underneath you. Comfy? Okay, plunge away. You'll barely notice I've left the premises.

I can see our little future clearly now. The fact that I'm too much for you. Are my mental processes, my complex symptoms too scary? That's surprising with your credentials, but undeniable given your way of ignoring parts of me. You work hard to steer me away from anything that hints at madness, and then redirect my attention towards filling up a social calendar. Just look normal, just act normal... oh, babe I've heard it all my life.

"You don't talk much about what you do at work..." Your revolting remark from last Thursday. What I do at work is meaningless, and has nothing to do with who I am. And if I tried to tell you that, you'd only smirk and shake your head. We know each other now. Can predict that we won't like what we'll see. In this past month, it's become clear that where we're headed together is only where we've already been. Such a shame Cleo's dead. She would've loved you, doctor. You're one and the same. I've wasted two years worth of money on a therapy that I got for free as a child. *Just tell yourself you're okay.* There. Now feel better?

Is That All There Is? Lyrics and vocals by Miss Peggy Lee.

Otis talked about that song a lot. He thought it neatly summed up the whole of life. But Cleo said it was an awful song, because no one should be like that, no one should give in to being sad... Mary Jane liked listening to Peggy Lee because she was always so sexy and classy. Some people noticed she moved kinda slow like Peggy and was soft and sensual. On and on and on. Yeah, well, it kept us dancing....

I've started having great fantasies at work lately. There's a large elegant bathroom on our floor, and when nobody's around, I can sit on a small sofa by the mirror and just think. If Connor worked in a place like this, well, clearly Jack would think it was doomed to fail. She'd hate it of course, but it might be fun to stay there just to irritate him. Sometimes, he thinks he understands her, and that's the ultimate joke.

Jack	*I can't read your mind, Connor.*
Connor	*Wow. Well that certainly clarifies everything. Gee, maybe I imagine things. Wait, oh, this is just a thought...but maybe just maybe I'm fucking INSANE!*
Jack	*Annoying, yes. Insane, no way.*
Connor	*Then why am I in this goddamn hospital?*
Jack	*Excellent question.*
Connor	*To keep me out of the way. Time's up. You're dismissed.*

Jack	We have a few more minutes. Do you think I'm in a hurry to get away?
Connor	I would be.
Jack	Maybe, wait, oh, this is just a thought...but maybe, I'm a nicer person than you.

He likes her so much, and it's clear she can't let herself see that. So they fight, always. He fights because it's the way she likes to communicate while she does it to save her very life.

"What about romantic relationships?" Strauss on a very bold day.

"I've told ya. No interest. Never had any." I have my own mind, okay? Leave me alone.

"You'd like me to think of you as asexual..." Yes, I would because you might stop wasting our time.

"I've had sexual thoughts at work, okay?"

"About who? Someone there?" When will I get it through my head that you just aren't listening at all?

"You feeling okay?" Elaine asks when I come back to my desk. "You were in the bathroom a long time..."

"Yeah. Guess it was something I ate. I'm fine now."

Jack	Don't throw away this chance, Connor. Work with me!
Connor	I'm right here for god's sake.
Jack	Yeah, you and all your smart remarks.
Connor	BLACK, said the pot.
Jack	Sarcasm has its place. There's more though. More to talk about.

She stands up and heads for the door, and he grabs her arm. Always the contact. The anger. Masking something. Something else. She knows he hates her. He has to. Who wouldn't? She wants a different doctor...

49

Talking about closeness and caring and Casey's recent boyfriend pain. I took a couple of days off from work to be with her, to console and remind her that she'll find the right guy, she will. Rescuing behavior. Caring too much. I don't want to change how I am with her. Yes, I give too much, but it's the only part of me that's good. There's got to be a redeeming hour in every life, one corner of a room not shadowed in loathing. I care more about Casey than I do myself. And because of that, I can endure who I am.

"I'm thinking of a scene in the movie you like, *Women In Love*. The young newlyweds at the picnic, remember? In the rowboat, she goes in for a swim, takes off her clothes...." I've seen it a dozen times. Her husband of less than two hours watches in horror, dives in after her. She can't handle the undertow, in an instant she's gone...he loves her, he loves her. All the wedding guests scream. He can't swim at all. But he loves her so he tries. Knowing he can't save her, he loves her, so he dies. "Then their two naked bodies wrapped in each other's arms, lying on the shore, right? Dead, in a lover's embrace." I hear you, and I know what you want me to glean from that moment. Casey and choices and a less arrogant therapist would call it co-dependency and use jargon befitting talk shows. But you're turning into quite the show-off, Poet-doctor, delivering your parable by describing my favorite art film. A doctor who chooses words that paint pictures. But there's ploy in it all, and don't believe for an instant that I don't see. Did you go rent the damn movie after I mentioned it? How else could you remember the details from fifteen years ago? I don't need you to do this, please. Don't dig around inside yourself to find a part that fits with me. Save it for someone who hasn't been loved, for some lonely little patient you can puff up and salvage, because I'm not in need of this. I did not come to you looking for this.

I criticize you all the way home. Still, the words stay with me – your words, not my own.

"Everybody who walks through these doors wants to feel better. But not one of them wants to change..."

"Of course I do. I do." A subtle nod. "Why else would I keep coming here, paying you, talking about this, if I didn't want to change?"

50

As if he was expecting that. "Lots of reasons." And eyes that smile.

Something very odd happened last night. Alone in bed, reaching only for my thoughts, the power of them, in the dark, unspoken images, smooth and soft and angry and hot...in thought, all paradoxes are allowed. Alone in bed, where wild things are, where a slap is a kiss, an angry word, a caress...anyway, anyway, while I was there in my mind not bothering a single soul, your words came in. And they almost sounded like Jack.

"You don't believe I want you to help me?"

That smirk. "Well... I believe you sure want me to *try*." No one has ever talked to me this way. What are you after?

I Do Not Come From A Long Line Of Changers

"Can't you see what's gonna happen, Mama?" Otis' face is contorted like a character from a Greek tragedy, and he holds her hand with both of his, imploring her. "It's inevitable! How can you not see?!"

She winks at her dear, thoughtful 60-year-old son. "It's okay, honey." She loves it when he holds her hand. "We just won't put any more on there..."

"Of course not! You can't let her." They stand together and stare at it. "Something has to be done, Mama. You can't let her just do whatever she wants."

"I'll take care of it, honey. Please don't worry."

"No, that's the last thing I want. You're an old lady, Mama."

"Oh, you're only old if you think so..."

"It could fall right on top of your leg and stick through a vein!"

"All right, honey. It's all right. We'll just leave it for now..."

The treacherous item under discussion is a narrow wooden table next to Mary Jane's living room chair. On the top she keeps her movie magazines, each one read from cover to cover, favorite pictures torn carefully out and placed in a smaller pile of their own on the footstool. Photoplay, Modern Screen, Hollywood Mirror month after month, placed on top of one another, the oldest touching the wall. About mid-way up the stack is where their problem starts. Slick paper and bent spines have formed an MGM Tower of Pisa, the top half angled in clear defiance of gravity. When Otis counted them that morning, he almost lost his breath. "A hundred and forty-two, Mama! She's got 142 of them waiting for you like a death trap!" His theory of the pending avalanche centers around how rapidly the books will likely slide, cascading across the floor before any human eye could be warned. He then sees Mama surrounded by colorful glossy banana peels, and being so startled by the noise, she'll whirl around with no safe place to put a foot. If the jagged corner of a Photoplay hasn't already poked one of the bulging veins above her ankle and splattered the movie stars' faces with gushing blood, she needs to consider herself "lucky beyond words" and remain perfectly still. But he fears she won't, that she'll try to walk through the slippery chaos and as plastic house shoe meets magazine centerfold, she will crash to the wooden floor and writhe in agony from her inevitable snapped bone. The picture he paints is so vivid and grisly that Mary Jane bursts into tears.

"I'm so sorry, Mama. Oh, I'm so sorry..." she gasps for forgiveness of an event that never happened.

"Honey, its all right. Otis is just saying things is all... We're okay..." Then he says more things, and although it's 6:00, no one is hungry because there's only worry in the air.

"Why'd he say that?" Mary Jane cries to Mama, in front of him, behind him, around him.

"I only said what is true," he turns to Cleo, looks into her for understanding, hoping she'll take his side "for once" and deconstruct the tower while there's still time.

"We'll always be all right," is the best she can offer. Then she says how lucky they are to have each other to care about, how some people are alone, but not them, no, they keep good watchful eyes on each other and Otis is so very cautious and such a wonderful man. He's the only man like that, she swears, and Mary Jane says that's true since she remembers the guys she dated and they weren't like that at all, only thought of themselves and what they could get. Otis says he tries to do good, wants to

always help out. "And you do!" Mama cries. "Every day!" We need one another. Life is filled with narrow tables and tall magazine stacks, and most people don't care, don't even notice let alone give a damn. Then Mary Jane remembers reading that very morning about a movie producer saying how funny it was that in Gone With The Wind when Clark Gable said "damn" at the end, it was such a big deal and the studio didn't want to let him say it but they went ahead and left it in because it was important to the story and now look at how much awful stuff they say and do in the movies when all poor Clark Gable was doing was just trying to say his line. Times have changed, they say. And not for the better, no not for anyone's better and to think how hard it was on the poor old movie stars who had to dress and talk a certain way all the time. They weren't appreciated, were they, those __real__ stars who had such rough lives. Lana Turner's daughter killed Lana's lover. It was in all the news. How horrible, how awful. Things were hard for all those stars, but maybe things are harder now in a way, tough to say, but it's certainly very different and really not for the better.

Mama asks if they're hungry and Mary Jane says yes and Otis won't eat if its gonna be any trouble, but no trouble at all and it's meat loaf, too. Good for a sandwich later if he's not hungry now, but he says he'll eat, he'll do whatever's easy, and TV trays come out and there's bread on a plate and some good mashed potatoes ("don't use so much salt" "there's bacon in with the beans so be careful" "that tray leg is wobbly" "don't use so much ice...") Maybe tomorrow they'll move a few magazines off the stack, but Mary Jane's not really ready, still needs to cut out a few pictures she saw, and Otis will help her to find them, can help her sort through them, but it could be too hot in the morning and the mail might come early... Mama says not to worry. Just eat and relax and figure something out later. No need to keep thinking cause we'll leave it for now.

The human personality is designed to stay the same over a lifetime. It builds on top of character that is set like concrete during childhood. The longer we live, the more entrenched we become – in what we like, what we fear, and the specific ways we avoid anything imagined to be unpleasant or threatening to our well-being. Structural change is more than *hard* – it violates the mind's stability. If it were easy, if we *weren't* wired to maintain status quo with such ferocity, we would all go mad. Lacking a reliable ground of being, a frame of "sanity" through which to filter all choices and perceptions, we'd sway with the slightest provocation. We'd be so open to novelty, there would be nothing dependable at all. But by nature's design, we become so "fixed" in ourselves that we can easily reject or ignore any stimulus that doesn't concern us, i.e. doesn't fit into the schism we know ourselves to be.

"Reject." "Reject," We fire back daily at bombarding possibilities. "Tilt." "Accept." "Reject." Me. Not Me. Not part of the solid rock I've built. That's the challenge of the "Talking Cure" with therapist as woodpecker, tapping away at damned *hard* wood, confronting conclusions, interpreting unconscious connections and trying to highlight what might be better handled from a different approach. Often a patient agrees full-out, affirming "yeah, definitely! Change would be great! That's a much better perspective, doc." But little change actually happens. If any at all. Tap tap chip chip. The wood is like steel.

However, there are turning points when something new can actually occur. The surface crack is instantaneous. A shift offers an opening, nothing more -- just enough of a quake to allow potential resettling on different ground. Of course, it may resettle back to the same way it always was. No guarantees. But against better odds, the *possibility* for change has occurred – and is undeniable.

Thursday 6 p.m.

"I guess I don't understand how this process is supposed to go..."

"You're not doing it wrong."

"I've told you what happens in my mind...I keep trying to explain it better..."

"No, you've explained it very well." An odd pause and he shakes his head. "A lot of times people think if they can just describe their symptoms, so the doctor can understand...then the *doctor* can fix things..."

"Okay, I get it. But then what...?"

"We've been talking lately about areas in your life you might want to look at differently. Try to see from a new perspective..."

"So you point out what I should change, and that's supposed to work?"

I haven't gotten such a big laugh in weeks. "No, that doesn't seem like its gonna work for you." Amazingly, you swear that for some it does. A suggestion here, a prod there, and Obedient Loony is off changing, trying new ways. Amazing. But other people require empirical proof – needing to grasp from the inside out just why they think the way they do, what secondary gains are savored. "Some people flat out won't be told what to do." At least we understand each other.

Mary Jane was working as a cashier at the Saengar Theatre the year Minsky's Burlesque came to town. Old Mr. Minsky thought she was just the prettiest thing he'd seen in very long time. "You could have been in his show." Cleo reminded. "He would have put you on the stage, you know..." Oh, she knew. Of course, Mr. Minsky was a little blinded by her breasts and hadn't noticed the paranoia. It wouldn't have been one of his better choices. Luckily, Mary Jane had her own reasons for saying 'no.'

"Yeah, he sure liked me, all right." She smiled exactly like Betty Grable. "And that was somethin,' all right. But you know me, I didn't want to have to dress a certain way and act a certain way. Those showgirls aren't frcc. I ncvcr could stand anybody telling me what to do."

"That's right, honey" Cleo said. "You always had a mind of your own." Truer words there are not.

PART TWO

Monday, 5:00 p.m. appointment.

FINALLY, a rating of Five Stars (and 2 Thumbs Up) for *a fascinating, entertaining, and ultimately harrowing session.*

Maybe I should just face that life *is* film (that apple falling close to the topiary schizo and all). Came into the session very playful today. Excessive amounts of valium will make a child too frisky. A new Woody Allen picture, *Husbands & Wives*, opened yesterday, and I went down to 84th Street to catch it last night. And, fuck us all, so did somebody else. It takes him three quarters of the session to bring it up.

"I'm wondering why you haven't mentioned last night…" What? "It's up to you, of course…" What? "But *not* mentioning it has meaning, too…" *What*??? Seems as I was coming out, he was waiting to go in (boy, that fits). It also seems I looked right at him and didn't respond. Swearing with every fiber of my unconscious, I did not see the man.

"Of *course* I would have said hello" I do not like this.

"You wouldn't have had to…" Not one bit.

"I would have wanted to… I have no idea why I didn't see you. Maybe Casey and I were talking…could you tell?

"Actually, I didn't see Casey at all. I thought you were alone."

"She must have been walking right next to me."

"I was focused on you…" I shake my head, and he immediately says we don't have to talk about this now if I don't want. (thought I was trying to "shake" you off? Connor laughs when Jack says that kind of shit).

Then I start to "replay" it, this imagined memory. As if *we* are the movie now, I see a long shot of the lobby, so many people all crowded together. Pretty cool people, too – the upper West Side intelligentsia that always come out for Woody. Cut to a medium shot of the good doctor standing with other cattle behind their rope, faces watching faces to see if the departing viewers

56

look satisfied. I wear a blue jean shirt over dark leggings, but then it's Connor, becomes a game-thought and she's being seen by Jack. He focuses on what, symptoms maybe? I can't remember if I did anything odd in the lobby, but so what, who cares. Long shot again, Jack's face following hers. No! This has nothing to do with Connor, …get out of my goddamned head. She'd say that, I guess. She'd be purely pissed. And for my own two cents, you can spy on me at the movies, you can follow me around this goddamn city if you want to, but you cannot come into these thoughts.

"What just happened?" he leans forward. Go away.

"Nothing."

"You rolled up your sleeves just then…I wondered if you were angry," kind of chuckles. "Maybe ready for a fight?" I laugh, too. It's fine, of course, all is fine. This is pure silliness, his words remind. Safe. Sterile. And dull. All is fine.

"Or maybe I was rolling them up to go to work," I offer, and he laughs out loud.

"You're so quick…" Oh, stop it. We sit in quiet. "What are ya thinkin?" You've studied it all, haven't you? From Freudian drives to Lacanian signifiers, through the wheat of Winnicott's good enough Mom to the chafe of Harry Stack's object obsessions. While I talk, your mind is so busy sorting through surface to depth and deciding who's projecting what identification onto whom that you must feel like a hard-working genius. You probably are, sweet boy. Just bear in mind that I'm thinking the same and then some. Alongside my self-reflecting searches for metaphors to baffle or entertain you, I'm also spinning tales of dominance games and alluding to quantum references and watching for signs of Revealing violence while playing a track about Connor, sifting through words dull as coal for any nuggets worth saving for late-night thinking, and all the while I'm watching you watching me and evaluating how invested you seem. So pardon me if I'm not quick to answer when you ask, "What are ya thinking?"

"Honestly, last night, I simply didn't see you." A friendly smile.

"Well, okay," and a suspicious pause. "The movie, though – it *was* about *couples*…" God bless a horse so dead it's decomposing. At least he's got the good taste to grin through this diatribe. "In fact, mostly very *troubled* couples…"

Without fully realizing it, my mind goes to Jack. "You mean, like couples who can't ever *agree*?" As I ask, my voice is a little too loud, too taunting for me. "Where no matter how much one protests, the other refuses to hear it?" He laughs hard and looks into my eyes.

"Oh, methinks this Lady doth protest a bit *too* much." I don't understand where we are these days. The only thing that could explain it is if you somehow knew about Connor, and that is absolutely not possible.

Then he looks to the clock - clearly a staking of power. The One who can end things. Oh really? Connor's a bit powerful too, I want to say. She has the power to never start. But back to us, back to the room. And suddenly I'm only angry that our time's up. Too much wasted on this crap, and we couldn't get around to my realization about feeling more anxious in the summer, when it's hot, and that maybe blood vessels constricting…

As I start to open my mouth, he reaches back to the desk and picks up his calendar. *Now* what? Another vacation, probably. Just leave a back-up and all is forgiven. Even an unknown someone, as long as she/he's decent. Vouched for. In case of emergency, don't break your own veins. Suddenly, the calendar is back on his desk and he's almost standing. "Okay, then. I'll see ya Thursday…"

"I uh, thought you were gonna tell me, or ask me something…"

"Nope. Just checking an entry…"

I don't move. "Oh, please don't do this. I know that had something to do with me."

"Honestly didn't," he smiles. "I was just looking to see who was scheduled for the next appointment." I truly don't know if he's serious.

"While I'm still *here*?" My breathing changes. A lot changes.

"We were getting ready to stop for today…"

"But we hadn't stopped. I don't know. I don't understand why you did that."

"I'm not sure what it is you think I did. We can talk more about it on Thursday…" The everything's-okay smile. The lie. "If you want to…

It's not what I *thought*… See me. See what's happening here… But he wants me gone. The hour is clearly up now, and he gestures to the door. A flimsy nuance. An intimation. I know what you *want*. He just nods, and looks so pitifully helpless. If you want me gone, *point*! Just walk over there like a fucking *man* and open the door and push me out! Have the decency to own it.

But I say none of that. As I leave, I'm not even sure what's true, or what only seemed to happen. On the street I feel like it was real. It feels. And that is no guarantee. I should wave for a cab, but only stand there. Waiting for him, knowing he's bound to realize… he'll think of how I looked, and know what happened in there. It's not out of the question for him to understand what he did, and come out here after me. He could realize how disorienting that was for me, see how he upset me and come out to see if I'm here. He could do a lot of things. In ten minutes a cab stops without provocation. How ambitious people are at first. Before I met Strauss, he returned my call within the hour. We kept missing each other (how prophetic) but he called back three times, sounding concerned, sounding responsible -- enough to make me choose. In the cab, the driver says it's gotten windy, and I nod. His I.D. photo reads "Michael Juarez." His face is the wrong face. Don't keep chatting at me, Michael. Don't grin and ramble because you think I want it. Right now your tip is less than a dime. "You're pretty harsh about other people." Words of the doctor. "you know how everyone is…" words of dead grandmother. Not that I could care if I tried. The slippery teachings, the lies the shit the party line and it's no party you'd be caught dead at but just like Michael Juarez, doctors ramble and do not listen… "you seem to have a very narrow view of people." Shut the fuck up and face what I already know.

Back at work, I can barely think. "Are you okay?" The omnipresent Elaine. (Go away, all of you, Mary Jane and Otis and anyone else who knocks on the bedroom door). I did not imagine what Strauss did, that much is clear. He played with reality, doing the one thing I told him makes me crazy. Unexpected. Off-kilter. Cli-click… it was purposeful. To test me or to show me it means nothing? Orchestrated for someone's benefit and maybe mine.

Rigged. Of course. But I have to know, to hear him say it - and not three days away. I have to understand the rules on the box if we're gonna play with these dice. He must know I'm gonna call because that's part of it, has to be. To see if I'll take care of myself and ask him again what it was about. I dial, still angry, mostly scared. Too new, this approach. Whatever he's trying, he's trying…. See me tomorrow? Make time for me? "I'm not handling this new tactic of yours well at all."

"What? What tactic?" Of course. Queen's Knight to Pawn-four. The game continues. My mind is distinctly cold. Ice crystals. As if cells inside my skull are changing. A DNA trigger has gone off, and there might be crystals forming where neurons have been. It could indeed be a changing of the Poles. Resulting needlessly in so much death. Something has gone terribly wrong. There's not an imbalance or there is…I can't even think! And it's none of my doing. I did not cause this and I did not see it coming! Every "crazy" state I've ever been in feels like a *game* compared to this. What in God's name have you done to me?

The next night he's there. Willing to see me. And so it is. I haven't slept and for whatever reason, I apologize for that. "This is a *good* thing that happened," he says softly. "…for us to see how upset you can get when you feel wounded." I'm incredulous. He denies over and over that his sin was intentional. Not a ploy. Not technique. Not anything.

"I've told you that reality shifting, something totally unexpected …I can't take it. That's what brings on that state…" He barely listens without even *trying* to pretend.

"No. I think you were very hurt by me. Feeling "unreal" is a way of protecting us." He says more. Keeps going farther and farther away. We're lost at sea now. Diverged. I try to stay with you. Not saying thoughts, not feeling the pain of being so misunderstood.

"No." I manage. One last arm above the waves before going under. "That's not me at all."

"It probably doesn't feel like you. That's what defenses *do*…" I nod. It's all there is left to do. Nod in disagreement.

So dark outside. It's the first time I've been in this room so late. The lamps are more golden, colors in the rug have gotten deeper. It's a different world this late. Could mean all bets are off.

"I know you're still very angry. You can say so if you want." Slight smile. Of course you'd smile. You're no longer looking at me. "...can say anything you choose..." Okay, then I will.

"Maybe since I've been hard to understand, you've literally tried to turn me into somebody else..." My hands are shaking.

"No." No smile at all. "Exactly the opposite." I can't look up, not even to check the time. There's little left to see. It's clearly the Ice Age. The shifting of the Poles was a random act, but that didn't make it any less disastrous. There is no one. None who have understood. This is not some harmless banter. Never has been.

"Something has gone very wrong. Something is happening... there are things about me you don't know."

"You can tell me..." I nod. And we all know what that means.

"I'm sorry, but I can't take this. I'm getting worse..."

"No. It might feel that way...different emotions are coming to the surface..."

"...it's more than I can take..."

"We're not in any hurry here. Always, we go at your pace..." It has all been playtime up to now. Inside my head, I'm shrieking. But there's no one to hear. Coming into this room was the biggest mistake of my life. He looks at me, not hearing the screams. Not seeing how little of me there is left.

"I'm suggesting we examine this relationship – between you and me, because it's right here in front of us. And from that, you can extrapolate out. We're in the middle of something here. Part of you knows it – and wants to run away."

"I'm not running anywhere. Things are just not what I thought. I had tried so hard to feel safe here."

"But now you don't."

"Please, it's not your fault. I thought I'd told you. You must not have seen it the way I was trying to explain..." We talk. Keep talking. I have no idea what we say. All that matters is that I was beginning to think you understood. For over a year I've been growing sicker, and we neither one saw. Both of us living in

61

delusion about who you are. From the time I walked in here, saying how troubled I am and how careful we need to be, and it could get worse. You said it wouldn't, and I asked again, and you nodded over and over...and said you'd stay here and listen. Well, I bought it. Hook, lies and thinker, until I finally woke up and saw that no one was listening at all.

Let it go now, okay? We did what we could together. Helped me for awhile. Let me go.

Please, Cleo! Help me. The world moved.
No, honey. You're okay...We're all right here.

Connor	*Do you want to hear it? How fucking crazy I really am?!*
Jack	*What I want is to try to help.*
Connor	*You smug, self-righteous son-of-a-bitch.*
Jack	*I am not your enemy, Connor.*
Connor	*Prove it.*

"It's more than anxiety," I whisper. "Always has been. I just didn't want to go into it..." Is this a typical event, Sir Strauss? Patient holds back and one day comes in announcing you never had a clue. In my case there's almost too much to choose from. Pick a symptom. I may describe how I used to cut myself up. Slice into my legs because it seemed to appease... or I might talk about the revolting things I let them do to me at Lara's. No. You might enjoy that one. I could talk about the tinkering kind of thinking and how it's every bit as crazy as my mother's, and we all see what happened to her. "I've let you think it's just panic attacks...like racing heart and a feeling of fear...it's much more" He tries to listen. But he's too defensive now to really hear. So I settle on cutting. It's in all the texts, so the shock won't be too much for him and isn't a sign of real madness. Serious enough, but not so bad as to put my autonomy in danger. "and used to hurt myself all the time. Stick things into my own skin. From the time I was little, haven't in so long. But wanting to. Again. Can feel that I'm falling, maybe all the way down.."

"How young were you? When you cut yourself?" Look at that. He's taking notes again. "It's always been clear that there's deep pain beneath what you show the world. And the more you tell me, the more I understand..."

Anyway, things are different now. You got that? Or maybe you can't tell, yet. Maybe you don't realize you asked for me, brother. Well, I'm fucking *here*.

"And, like you said, needing to try to hide it, you know..."

"Even from your psychiatrist." He looks concerned. The room is a deeper golden as if someone's changed the bulbs. There's a new smell, like an incense-sandalwood, something musky. His eyes are darker, and that gray turtleneck doesn't look like what he was wearing when I came in. Reality is different, but it's not The Revealing. Not this time. We should have stopped though. Oh, dear God, I shouldn't have let you keep talking.

"You imagined that if you were 'good' – if you only told me the barest essentials, then one day I'd fix everything?" Yes. "Like with your grandmother." But I *had* told you, or so it seemed. Maybe I never actually said it in words, but I thought it so often, and I knew you'd see when you were ready. "I can't read your mind," you say it kindly and a little sad. Is that what you meant every time you said it? Telling me that you really couldn't see? I only listen. "Protecting us, in a way. Just showing me the tip of the iceberg..." Cli-click. Strands of icicles that I can see in his hair. Does he realize what he said? Impossible. No one could be that slick.

And with that, total awareness.

"What's happened?" he leans forward. "What are ya thinking *right* now?" Tears. And thinking only that you're a good man, a very gentle one. I was wrong to imagine you might be tricking

63

me. It's clear that you're no part of it. Not at all. You're being used without your knowledge. The words were put there without agreement. None of this was your fault. But you weren't strong enough to stop it from happening.

"I'm sorry I got so confused…" The tears won't stop.

"No, no. It helps us to understand…." Diverged. North was South and no one saw it coming.

Cleo, where are you? I need to go!

"You're wrong," I nearly whisper. "You don't get it at all." I'm so sorry.

"Then tell me more – so I *can* …" Why now? All this warmth now when it's too late… the irony is excruciating. "You're not alone here, okay?"

Oh, yeah, I know. That's what's so goddamn terrifying.

Delusions R Us

Ordinary feelings and simple thoughts – that's what delusions are made of.

"You'd like it to be much more complicated." He adds. Of course. Mad women are exotic creatures, doctor. Mysterious, paradoxical. Beyond reach. *"There's* the important phrase!" You're right.

So another blow to my ego as you insist that my unconscious mind is not some elusive, brilliant enigma destined to confound us all. I want my money back.

Simple feelings. Those are the culprits? Dangerous thoughts perceived as unacceptable, but no matter how hated and feared, cannot be willed away. So as protection, the mind invents a disguise where emotions (real as wool) can hide in sheep's clothing. The lamb of madness.

Rage at a loved one? A world war breaks out.

Murderous jealousy?   My skin turns strange colors and monsters stare from the shadows. (yep, that green-eyed one). The Unconscious is a shameless comedian prone to very bad puns.

The doctor seemed kind and caring, but when he looked at that calendar, ignoring me, leaving me while I still stood right there... The disappointment was unbearable. In the most literal sense of that word. My Protector is dead. The man I was almost starting to need, I now hate. Welcome to a Shifting of the Poles. In a language of symbol and metaphor, North becomes South. Good is evil. Nothing is what it was, and no one is safe. The world itself can be destroyed by my ambivalence. And if I am that powerful, paranoia is a mere survival tactic. So coincidental happenings suddenly have great meaning. The word "iceberg" is prescient.

Then I look into his face and the next revision is created. He seems sad, as if he cares deeply that he hurt me. So it doesn't look like world destruction after all. Touched by the kindness in your eyes, disarmed by the kindness, I'm back in the room, it's just you and me again. For you with the warm expression, I'll make you powerful. I'll weave us both an excuse by discovering that what you did was a trick. That's the only acceptable answer. Solution to my convolution. You are not bad or careless. You really are brilliant and created a trick for my own ultimate good, setting me up, I played along as I should, and any minute you can come clean. You'll tell why you did it, explaining a technique designed to improve my lot, never to hurt me. I'm sorry I didn't have enough faith and couldn't see the warmth for all the ice.

But you deny it, refusing my gracious offering of an "out," so again my delusion gets re-written. Now you're not a Master Wizard with secret techniques. In your stead is left only a man, a flawed listener, a doctor who just fucked up, one of those ordinary humans with repulsive transparent seams. I feel enormous rage - of supernatural potency and realize you're nothing. Just a poor guy being *used* by Powers beyond us both.

Remarkably I'm feeling stronger.

The truth behind this fantasy is that he *has* been duped - all the things I've kept secret, thoughts intentionally held back. Then with great relief, I see there's been no supernatural power at all, and I write the last chapter of the fantasy. It's only I who've been using him. My sad would-be caretaker was pawn to a queen. Filled with sympathy now, I look into his eyes and smile. The man has done nothing terrible because I've been in control all along. And that one I can live with.

"You don't have to pretend its okay," he tries again. "You can *tell* me that you're angry..." I gently shake my head. Don't be silly. At this point, I don't feel a shred of anger. None at all.

-     *Cleo, tell me a story, please.*
-          *Honey, you know I'd do anything for you.*
-          *Oh, yeah. I sure do.*

"I need some Stellazine," Finally something of value gets spoken, but *you* should've said it. I'm getting so goddamn tired protecting you. "Some of the books I read – and I know you don't think it's helpful for me, but I already did, okay? There's no good pretending I don't know what I know..." I stop to breathe, to sneak in a very deep breath, not wanting it seen or analyzed. "I've read that some people get worse in treatment..." He nods slowly.

"That's true, unfortunately." Am I relieved or saddened? Is he? One or the other and no idea which..

"That's what's happening," I say softly. "It's not your fault, you couldn't have known. The kinds of thoughts I've had lately, they're a sign to stop." He listens, frozen. Envious perhaps, that I'm the one with the courage to bring it up. "I don't mean a "sign" in a paranoid way," I smile, but get nothing back. "This whole process is too much for me. I haven't been completely honest, but it's making me *crazier*." Still nothing. "We need to call it quits."

"Is that what you want?" (Didn't I just *say* that?) "You're still so angry at me that you need to think about leaving. I realize I really hurt your feelings, although I didn't mean to at all."

"Why do you keep *saying* that? My god, nobody gets psychotic because somebody hurt their feelings!"

"Oh, yes. Some people most certainly do." It's a victory to him, a blow successfully landed. "I'd like to take a guess at what went on with you. Okay?" Sure. A guess. I do like the honesty. "I did hurt your feelings, and what surprised ya wasn't that I made a mistake, that I was clumsy. That's nothing new, right?" A mutual smile as anchor in some raging sea. "It surprised you that you cared. That you *could* be hurt by me at all. That this relationship matters that much," and he laughs. "Or maybe at *all*." I nod, and with it, with agreement on this shameful topic I feel like I'm literally disappearing. I am not playing at all right now. And the wheel is turning and no one is at any helm. "Look, if I suspected that you were getting worse here, I'd encourage us to talk about it. That's not what's happening with you." Silence. So much icy silence.

"I don't understand what it is you want me to do…"

Wearing his best kind smile again, "You do keep trying to figure that out. I really don't have a secret plan."

Cleo, why does everybody lie?

"But what if I want to quit? It's my decision."

"Of course it is. And if you'd choose to stop coming here, I wouldn't be angry at you. Certainly it would be your decision. However, I don't think it would be a very good idea." Plu-perfect and future perfect… advanced English grammar is an important subject for a good psychiatrist. His words about my potential decision come from a nether-world of hypothetical tenses. Not "*when* you decide" not "I *won't* be angry," – but "*if* you were to… I *wouldn't* be…" Don't want any careless grammatical signals pushing me out the door. So diligent. But only when he feels like it.

"Let me tell ya what I see." For half the session, revealing who you believe me to be. Cautiously, please. (Although it is exquisite torture). "Maybe what you *can't* do is continue like you've been. Maybe if you choose to stay here, you're saying something will change – not from me, but from *you*. And I think part of you wants that. Another part would do anything to prevent it."

We sit in silence for awhile. Peace. "And one more thing…" My god, right as you're standing up, ready to end the session. Why do you fucking *do* this?! "I also think, no, I know that if I had quietly accepted you wanting to leave your treatment, if I'd said '*okay, it's up to you, bye,*' you would have been very, *very* hurt."

In the park under beautiful autumn trees. A long shot. A perfect movie still. But for my ugliness in the frame. Close up on my hands, clenching, unclenching. Shaking, flinging themselves, no, I fling them as if they're wet. Get off of me! In my pockets, just put them away, hide them and pack them down. ("that something in *you* is changing…") Orange and yellow leaves close enough to touch. If, of course, I could use my own hands.

Cleo, can you come? Please!

He called it. Named it. I care what he thinks of me, this man, this doctor. As if shreds of fantasy games have bled into this room. But it's not real. Can't be.

No one gets to me. Not really. And no one ever will.

"…thinking that if you choose to stay, you can't continue as you have been…" Of course you're right. And I doubt you know how much.

"So if I can *tell* more about my past, more things I couldn't say…that would make the feelings stop?"

"That's part of it," he says. "Telling things. What also works is to examine this relationship here, between us." He wants me gone. Wants me to stop whatever I've been like with him. "To put it bluntly, up to now we've both shown a mutual respect for your facades.." The smile is kind, the words so mean.

Even if I wanted you to know me, it couldn't happen. Not someone like you. Won't happen, and it's dangerous to even try. And still, I just stare at you, amazed. No one has ever said anything like that to me.

"I *don't* wear a façade with you…" I offer. I've tried not to, anyway. I think. "I'm comfortable here. I trust you very much."

"Oh, *really?*" My God. "I think maybe you trust me a *little tiny* bit." He doesn't look afraid at all. "*Maybe.* But I bet it scares you that you *want* to." Treatment is a seduction. Don't ever believe otherwise.

I heard it over and over at Lara's from my regular clients. "You really understand me…" Yeah sure. Whatever.

"For you," Strauss has never been this talkative. I caused something, or he did. We did. "…trying to control other people by being what they want and letting them *think* you're more connected than you really are, it's a pervasive part of you. It's part of your character structure, and it doesn't serve you. It actually stops you from being able to have the real relationships with people that you can only have if you're not hiding emotions from yourself."

"I *don't* hide them from *myself* though."

And then very gently, "I disagree."

You want to see me as some kind loving child. It's a mistake. Please beware. I've never tried to lure you. Someone needs to stay strong, and yes, I protect you. I do it for me.

"You try to convince people you're above it all," he talks and I look into his rug. Watching lines and swirls that mimic a brain, electronic movement, faster than mercury. Weaving into pictures, then slipping apart. Analyze this one, quick. Before it fades away.

"…you pretend not to care what they think of you, that you don't really need anyone… and sometimes you *believe* it, and your pain seems to go away. But when that illusion gets punctured, you're aware of the pain again. Lately you've seemed so desperate about telling me things – you can tell me next week, or next month, or six months from now. We'll work on this as long as it takes – for you to be able to form different kinds of relationships, to realize that you can *matter* to someone – besides your family. Now later on, you'll likely suspect you *duped* me into saying all this – but ya didn't!"

69

How superior I've felt to you, and I wonder if you've had a clue. Can you hear this without hating me more? Yes, you're the one with M.D. near your name, and the one with the fine collectibles. A Persian rug doth not a great man make. Up until recently, you seemed *simple* to me, as if you were half a person. Nice, not bad at *all*, but lacking somehow. Like everyone.

"Seeing people as objects, as cartoon cut-outs..." (well, only when they *are*. But I wonder about you now. If you're as smart as I am, as aware as I am...)

"As *real* as you are, maybe?"

No one has ever come in this far. I'm not even sure how much of it is actually happening, or where Jack and Connor start and stop.

"Yes, there are things I haven't told yet," I'm being too bold. "But they're not secrets kept from me. I don't see how saying it all out loud could make a difference. I mean, isn't that right? It's the secrets we keep from *ourselves* that make us sick. A mask known to be a mask..."

"Maybe there are things you both know, and don't know..."

"Well, I certainly know how the mind works..."

"You say that a lot..." He looks so serious. Threatened? Not enough room in here for two experts. Shut the fuck up, I hear in myself. For once in your goddamn life, stop it. Then he leans forward, arms on knees, and all seriousness is gone from his face. It's as if he can tell how mean I am inside. As if, but not actually so. "Listen, I know you're smart, okay? And you probably have learned a great deal from what you've read. You've done well in the "Lecture Series" part. But what you've been missing is the *Lab*."

Something is completely different in you. Since the night from the movie and seeing me when I couldn't see you back...you've become someone else. What did you read in me that night that made you change?

The Stellazine lands on my emotions like a heavy tarp and within 24 hours I'm calmer but still bewildered. He's maneuvered me into wanting to divulge more, using some analytic trick I don't recognize... "I don't use tricks here." I will never understand.

    For the next few days I obsess over what I need to say. If ever, if ever I am to tell, it's probably now. Probably him. I think. Or not at all. I don't know and certainly don't know what good it could do. In the midst of it, I keep thinking of the 1940s headline "Garbo Talks." That was a hell of a year for Mary Jane. The entire country was excited along with her – "Talkies" were bringing to life the voices of Hollywood's stars. Beauties and hunks who'd been adored as images would now be heard as well as seen. And the loudest hype was over the vocal chords of Greta Garbo, darling of the silent screen. Someone that gorgeous would have to sound great or it'd be scandalous. Mary Jane was at the New Orleans premiere in the Loew's State theatre, even got her picture in the paper standing in the lobby filled with hundreds of fans...right in the center was Mary Jane wearing a wide black and white hat, tight red sweater, hip cocked to one side. She must have been a photo journalist's dream. And the surprise, always, of that tiny dainty face, a cameo perched on a street walker's body. "It was the most exciting night of my life." For 25 years, old newspaper photo stayed taped on the wall next to Rita Hayworth, another yellowed copy mounted in the kitchen. In time, I guess everyone gets their McCluhan Fifteen Minutes.

    In the lobby, there had been a couple standing near her, and the woman kept repeating what Mary Jane had read in Photoplay. What if Ms. Garbo didn't sound good at all? And what was worse, the woman acted like she actually *wanted* Greta to sound bad.

    It wasn't out of the question. Some stars were losing their place ever since these Talkies were invented. Some of the men who'd been so dashing in silence were being exposed as shrill-voiced, or the ultimate kiss of death, effeminate. A few glamour girls were turning out to be nasal, or accented in a way that did not charm. *We love you, we want you, all we want is to hear you! Ugh, go away. We don't like you anymore.* For some, progress could equal death.

    But for the rest of her life, Mary Jane would be claiming credit for Garbo's continued success. Because as my mother stood in Lowe's lobby on the night of that premiere, she decided to use her lifetime prayer.

Cleo always told us that God can't answer everyone about everything (well, he wasn't Cleo, after all). She said that once in a lifetime a person could expect a completely answered prayer, and that it was fine to ask for other things along the way, but ya had to wait and really think on what one thing you'd need most in life. It was a crafty way to explain why He'd been ignoring us all those years, and the pressure of "only *One*, remember" was enough to keep a houseful of nervous wrecks from yelling a Wolf call for anything petty. Cleo's own mother had come up with the idea that god was a one-trick genii, and Cleo sold the concept with such conviction that we all assumed it was actually in the Bible. So that night as Mary Jane stood in the lobby of the Lowe's State, she knew not to take things lightly. Someone nearby frowned at her outfit, and she shrugged her shoulders and stuck her chest out even more. I know what they think, she smiled to herself. Everybody is ruined by their jealousy, just like they're jealous of Greta. And that is the evil that makes them all so goddamn mean. She listened as the nasty woman rambled on about how Garbo was foreign after all, so maybe we wouldn't even understand what she said when she talked, and she laughed, the mean woman did. So many terrible things in this world.

It's the hardest truth to handle, realizing that there are bad things all around and there's just so little anyone can do. We can hear, and we can see. That's the hell of it. We can identify the bad, but then we have to live with of it. That's the hell, Mary Jane thought to herself. Knowing, and then just watching.

She thought about it for a long time, as all those strangers stood close together while the press took more pictures and the excitement grew. And then she closed her eyes. Mary Jane had always prayed for the stars to be happy. She worried so much and their lives were so hard. It wasn't easy to look like that, she knew. She knew. And it was just too much when other people are out to hurt you. And with that, she offered up her prayer of a lifetime. *If I never ask again, dear God, I want this tonight. Just let her sound good. She's always been one of my favorites, and people don't know how it might kill her if she wasn't famous anymore. The movie stars all worry every day if somebody likes them, if somebody hates them. She's one of my favorites, please god, this is it. Just let Greta sound good.*

Years later, this woman, my mother, would be unable to sleep straight through any night. She had used her one prayer. It was done. She was at the mercy of the world.

Monday 7 p.m. It may be time.

A humanely warm glow from the lamp tonight. Your face looks permanent to me, as if it's been in this room and in my life forever. Cleo, forgive me. If I believed in any god, if I had one prayer, it would be only that. *Cleo, forgive me.*

"If I do go into all this," I say, "promise you'll stay with me on it. I mean, that you won't leave while we're right in the middle of something..."

"You know who I am" You offer gently. Don't be rough with me tonight because I really couldn't take it. "There is nothing you absolutely must tell me. You know that. We go at your pace." If your warmth is artificial, I don't even care. Keep being this nice even its totally fake. "I'm not pushing you. Not at all." Then tell me it'll be okay. Please, just a couple of lies a little while longer. "What's been happening here, and we've talked about this, is that part of *you* is doing the pushing. Both the urgency and the fear about telling things – it's all coming from you." I feel your eyes on my face like light, moving over skin quick as flame. Looking for what, you don't even know. But with me, staying on me, unafraid. Have you been this attentive all along and I never saw it? "We're just two people here, working together, doing the best we can..." Alone in the room we watch each other with no one pretending.

Cleo, I'm so sorry for what I made you do. He doesn't need to know this. Some things are not for anyone but us.

"Maybe *starting* to tell is the hardest part..." His entire body is a vigil to me. And then it comes. So innocent, as it always does, my guard down, feeling bold, and it comes. He has no idea of the sin he's about to commit. "I'm *sorry* you feel so alone here..." And with it, a look of hurt. More important than words, over these many months, it's been the eyes that betray him. He wants to help me and can't. My secrets have made him sad. And

73

done. In a wave. Of compassion. It was bound to happen. I will never even blame him, the man with the warmest eyes and heart-patterned sleeve. It all got to me when I wasn't looking. It can't be any of our faults we're this fucking weak.

"All right then," I hear my bitterness. Guess I shouldn't have started if I wasn't gonna put out. "Pick up your notebook there, doctor. Trust me, you'll want to write this one down." He doesn't move. Eyes stay on me, ears. I have never been more aware of another human being, but I keep talking - and talk till there's no going back. Still no writing, no analyzing. Only him.

In one of Cleo's favorites stories the Sun and the Wind have a bet to see which can get a man to take off his coat the fastest. The Wind summons up all its strength and blows against him, trying to rip the coat from his shoulders, but the man only clings tighter. Easy to resist gales of bluster. And the Sun? Not even a challenge. Impossible not to succumb to heat.

Hey, toilet training ain't easy. Little kids can't wipe themselves, okay? They're doing damn good to get it in the goddamn bowl. Can't clean themselves right. Might be too rough. That area is very tender down there. It needs a careful hand and a gentle towel. All done, okay ? All clean. No big deal really it isn't, it just *isn't*. It's part of taking care of a child. And year just turns into year. Ask Bo.

What comes out of my mouth are words that should never be told. When the Good Princess spoke, rose petals tumbled forth, but from the lips of the Bad One came only toads. What's falling from mine should show in your face, but it doesn't. Tonight must seem like a breakthrough. A benchmark of trust. How things seem. In reality, it is repetition, dear doctor. See, I couldn't bear to hurt my grandmother's feelings, and tonight I couldn't hurt yours.

Yes, I'm opening up – for all the wrong reasons. I'm bringing you into the bathroom with me, so you won't feel bad. In the name of human compassion. Always in its name.

It's happening all over again.

I was prepared to try, to open up, simply tell…but you took it from me. You played the lines I sneaked into your mouth, and you wore your role well. Letting Cleo possess you in a way. And what you see as our strides are footprints of my past.

"Are ya okay?" Nearly time to leave, he leans forward.

"Yeah, sure." A mask is a mask is a mask. I'll just redress here. I'll be fine.

"You know to give me a call if ya need to..." Oh, can't we all see that happening? You get paid to be here. I'm here. Off the clock phone calls are for other people.

It's night and I know not to look at the moon. Something has been left though, back there in that room. I've done something, started something that we had no right to do.

"I'll make plenty of mistakes here..." You said once. "and I'm human, so I may forget something you tell me, or misunderstand...but that doesn't mean you're not important or that I'm not paying close attention to everything you say."

We're out of control now, off and running with no restraint. This work you do is dangerous. You have no right to do this to people's minds. "I'm just an ordinary therapist, doing as competent of a job as I can..." But I couldn't hear it. So you land on my foot with one more error in judgment and, in the end, I can only wonder how badly I'll be crippled. If I can endure, you say I'll learn the dance of life.

On the corner of Broadway and 72nd, I stand near the kiosk and watch strangers. It's spring and people sit at outdoor tables, sipping drinks much slower than at other times of the year. Things change, seasons, life. But not really. In six months, we'll all bundle under down and scarves, and then six months after that, the restaurants open their doors and prop up plastic tables near the sidewalk. It may only look like change, this eternal loop. Then I glance up, as I intended when I stopped here. It seems to be literally puncturing the indigo sky, this white creamy orb. It is honestly not the same moon from twenty years ago. It can't be, because tonight I started something with another person that I never planned to do as long as I lived.

It's too late to care.

Just dim the lights and swell the music, because we're in it now – with the clumsy and blind leading the tango.

It's painful being around Casey these days, but damn near impossible to be alone. She is not the way I used to see her, and I can tell what's she's thinking of me. "How's it going with Dr. Strauss?" Maybe I won't talk to anyone ever again. Oh, almost forgot, my little friend, have I mentioned that since treatment began, I've been getting much worse? Like a house of cards, every lie comes tumbling down. She's not going to be a famous movie star. Dreams are dreams. And we wake up with rotting flesh.

It's been weeks since I masturbated. Connor doesn't even exist.

"I'm sorry to call, but I wanted to know if I could have an extra appointment if you have any times available. Tomorrow, maybe?" Look at that, I have a new master.

"These new feelings you've got coming up, it's nothing to be so scared of, okay? It means nothing except this is where you are in your treatment." Now I happen to know that when a patient says something is "only" this or "just" that, when a patient says "means nothing except..." then the doctor has been alerted to look for more. Much much more.

In movies, if a child is being touched in a way that's wrong, if someone, say just someone is violated...if maybe hands are cleaning a body that is not their own... if I was in the bathroom, say... if she was there, if we were there, together as always, if we were there and it was a movie, if it was...just if... there would be such emotional music, I know there would. Soft, haunting violin or atonal piano chords...oh, there *would* be music to accent it all. Dramatically, the lights would dim, might be shadows of golden on our eyes and bluish white on our flesh. If it was a movie, there would be Atmosphere, punctuation of every sight and sound, because out of respect for the incredible interaction, Reality itself would pay homage.

But in Life (that low-budget release) it's all so ordinary. No soundtrack, no filters or gels - just a moment like any other, a tired old medium-shot from a tedious angle in the same well-lit bathroom with insignificant dialogue, a touch, a wipe, a warm towel, then one that's damp, chatter chatter, business as usual, fingers along me, chit chat, a running faucet with the silly pipe noise, pat dry, flush, smiles, chatter chatter, door opens, more talk, such idle talk, all the way to the kitchen, petty talk. Not an ounce of intrigue. Not one special effect. Merely us being us on a regular day.

So if ya ever start thinking that things are just not right, if it keeps coming to your mind that the whole thing is rather incredible, don't bother looking around – Reality itself yawns at the routine. Look, ya did it yesterday, and the world didn't end. Finally, you'll realize there will never be a climax, or denouement, or swell of music. This ain't no epic opera, drama queen. This day won't offer you any raving, ranting spot-lit moment. Not a bolt in the fucking sky. This is daily life, my dear, and no one bats an eye.

It'll all keep happening. In such an ordinary way. That's precisely what will drive you insane.

You love illness, don't ya doctor? Lately you're wearing that delicate smile all through a session, head tilted, forehead crinkled as you lean in, showing how much you want to listen. It tames you, my sickness does. Stops you dead in your tracks. See? I'm bleeding. See? Now back off, please, and don't touch. I'm already cut.

Other people can't possibly feel this way. Words would have been written if they did, and I could have read them.

Other people do not feel within themselves every tiny subtle shift of mind. The suggestion that I tell how I feel is absurd. They can hear because they have ears. So does corn. Neither will have a clue what I'm saying.

These are times I believed would never be. Too much of what's inside me is coming forward, available to the rest of life. No going back. The most terrifying phrase in the English language.

77

I hear people and see them talking, but they are not there. Everything around me is nothing but my imagination. I have made up the world. I am imagining myself.

"Try going for a walk or talking to a friend..." Yeah, that'll fix everything.

But twice a week for a hour, I seem to exist. It makes no sense.

"Lately, you're not as guarded when you're here..." You look strange today. Your face, your body. Too bright. Too distinct. Too much. Some days you look like "other people", the ones on PBS. Grown-ups with large libraries and leather chairs. Like the ones who walk in academic halls. Not real people, really. I don't know. Ones who never look at me.

Some of the women at work must get up at dawn to put themselves together. It's like they have a staff of professional costumers and make-up artists living in their closets. But more fascinating than the question of *how* they look so perfect, is the question of *why*. For six months now I've tried to care, been religious about the game, letting Casey dress me up to be corporate and polished. All those cream-colored blouses and camel blazers are mine, not mine, me. Of me. It's a time-delineated illusion, of course, because I notice that after lunch, my "look" isn't holding up very well. These goddamn women go into the bathroom throughout the day and re-touch, re-apply, straighten and smooth themselves, taming their hair and their psyches into obedient order. I can't care, and I know that makes me odd. I can't even care about *that* anymore.

Elaine works in the office across from me, and she thinks I'm witty and nice and she likes to chat by the printer. Basically she's fine, someone less "corporate" to her core than the other automatons. Yes, I like her in a way. I'm letting a few more people into my life.

"I'm trying, okay?" But Strauss doesn't look convinced. "Went out to lunch with Elaine a few times. Walked around the bookstore with her, I'm trying, okay? Trying to make new friends."

"You say that like you're doing it for me." Well, duh.

"You said I should."

"Oh, no...I said it was curious that you didn't have more people in your life. I never said you *should*.

May I please see the box top again? I've forgotten the rules of this game.

The last few months have brought a very bold move on my part. While Casey's always been our only star, I've confessed to having my own thoughts of performing. She doesn't take well to it, of course. I pretend not to notice and enroll in an improvisation class. Strauss seems to think it's fine, no, that it's great. I'm entitled to get out on a stage myself. There's nothing wrong with it; I'm not doing anything *to her*. My own life doesn't harm someone else.

It feels like a waking dream, but one that's not frightening. I marvel at the fantasy of being in New York, going to rehearsals, talking with other actors about doing a small performance in the Village. Oh, lovely, somewhere near Lara's? In a way, I hope it is and I can use the same subway, eat at the same diner. Maybe I'll glimpse a ghost of myself there, sitting at that back booth the way I did in the Lara days. A ghost who'd marvel at what I've managed to become – and realize I'm doing it for her in a way. Even on bad days, she had hope, and I'd like to show her what we are, that it wasn't all in vain.

At any rate, I'm out of the wings for a moment in time, and the exhilaration in Strauss' eyes might be mine. Not sure. But I'm not doing this for *him*, only for those ghosts of me. *Look at me*, I want to say to strangers. *Look what we did! I'm living in the world.* And in the next breath, I would ask this of those strangers - why am I not totally well? I've turned around 180 degrees, and little has changed. If this step didn't fix it, nothing will.

Several very bad depersonalized nights, an entire two-hour performance where I thought I was dreaming. "It's only a defense...nothing more. It can't hurt you." Distanced from my very life. What's the point? "...protecting you from unexpected feelings..." Like what?! What is so goddamn horrific that I can't feel it?! "Not so horrific. It's the surprise itself that's feared. Thoughts that surprise the thinker. Feelings that surprise the heart. Pretty threatening for someone who's tried to be so totally controlled."

"I feel real here. With you." I say.

"Sometimes." He corrects.

"Most of the time. Really."

"And when ya don't? It's when?"

"When I feel scared of something, thinking maybe I should tell you..."

"Or if you're disappointed in me."

"Yeah. If you do something unexpected."

"When the person I am in your mind becomes more important that the person I am in this chair. Right? Ya see that one?" Yes. When you're not Jack. Or Cleo. Or anyone I've invented. "And when the real flesh and blood and *imperfect* me threatens your mental image.."

"I shut you out."

"You *try* to."

"And when I can't?"

"Yep. That's *exactly* where the trouble starts."

"How, in all seriousness, how can it ever change?"

"We're working on it," He smiles. "It takes time." I'm sorry. I know you're trying so hard with me. I'm so sorry. 'You had a month or more where ya said you felt *good*, remember? Not dreamlike at all..." Right. And it was true. But when I get like this I can't seem to remember ever feeling different. "...to trust that it's a time-delineated feeling..." So's life.

Changes within a Self herald danger to a mind. Identity at stake. *Major alert, organism going down.* Depersonalization. Makes a bit of sense.

It's not me.

Not real.

Not happening.

I'm dreaming.

I'll wake up and things will be as they were.

I am this. I am not that.

"That's an awful lot of control you're trying for there..." I know. But I used to do it! I lived like this and I know it worked! "How well?" Better than this!!!

I will not feel different without my consent.

The way I was as a child, in my house...that *cannot be me.*

The way I was at Lara's...I am *not the things I have done.* I can't be.

"Maybe it's a *part* of you..." Then I want to be dead.

This isn't happening.

I'm not awake.

I've never been real.

The world is a dream.

I do not feel.

Nothing is true.

"I'm thinking about a poem," he says gently. "It might be Shelley. There's a line that reads something like...

Body swayed to music

...how are we to know the dancer from her dance...

I recognize it instantly. That poem exists in my memory banks, like a book that's been waiting on a high shelf since I was fifteen. After school, I used to take the bus to Siler's Bookstore on

Canal Street. Even on the scariest of days, I could manage the ride and the store was a few feet from the bus stop. A small canopy with windows of poetry and plays. Inside it was dark, atmospheric, not fluorescent-lit. Narrow aisles, conserving space for the books themselves and library ladders that reached rafters. I wanted to live there, literally. And imagined on my best days that it might be possible. Even the shoppers were different, all looking like scholars. People who care about what the pages had to say. Because on those shelves were words that actually did mean something. At night, I'd read them to Cleo. Not that she always understood, not every word, but she loved hearing me read, and I pretended that I was reading to the strangers, the scholars, who were more interested in the words than in me.

"It's not Shelley, it's Yeats," I say. "I used to love that poem. This is really something…" I doubt you could know. Can't know. After such a long time, hearing someone think of it – in connection to me. "It's called "Among School Children."

Oh, body swayed to music, oh brightening glance.
How can we know the dancer from the dance?"

"Oh, it's Yeats?" He asks. "Okay." Both of us smiling. "See? I certainly don't know everything."

Quite the save, doctor. Just when I'm ready to give up on us, you ride in on that poetic white horse. And I am disarmed. My eyes reach like outstretched hands. Hold onto me. The only way we can. Hold the gaze.

The pattern in his rug, dark blues and golds swirl, and threads connect like dots…places to crawl and sleep. I imagine it's warm inside that rug.

These are not my feelings. It's a game and I don't even understand its purpose. Unless of course, I need to seduce you. That makes perfect sense, because then I honestly would be safe.

"What was your grandmother's marriage like?" Basically a non-event. Tedious. Like most things.

He fell out of love with her one day. She swears she saw it happen, the moment when he looked at her in the bright sunlight of a rational mind and decided she was nothing so special.

"Oh, it didn't really matter," She reassured. "I was never in love with him..." We don't fall in love, my family. However, we are very good conduits through which love can flow, albeit *one-way* currents. Through charm, or breasts, or legs or smiles, by hook or by crook, we can captivate when necessary.

"There is no one else like you," one of my clients at Lara's said every time he saw me. Yeah, well, hon, in truth, then there is just NO one. See, I'm not really like me, either.

Every year our house fell towards ruin a little bit more. Well, we were very busy, so there wasn't much time to dust. Cleo tried periodically, sweeping the hall and middles of floors. But whatever was lying under a bed, or piled in a corner simply stayed where it had landed. Boxes and bags of "things to sort through" rested in closets and crannies. Throw nothing away. It might have sentimental value. Life is cumulative, after all. Whatever we were, we still are, what we ever once did, we still do. You can add things on, if there's room, but cast nothing off. You could hurt somebody's feelings that way.

In a loving home, nothing ever gets outgrown.

Whatever did happen to Baby Jane?

Bo, Bath & Beyond

I didn't find out the full extent of It All till we had to move. I was seventeen, moments from graduating high school. Seems Cleo had managed to beg the landlord to let us stay till I finished. They were just going to make some renovations, and they needed it empty. It wasn't anything really, just that they didn't know what exactly they wanted to do with the house, and they needed it empty. Sure.

The fact that my mother hollered, my uncle occasionally walked in the street barely dressed, the fact that I was up all hours lately and the only way I could stay calm was to keep hiking up the T.V. volume as the night got darker... nooo, they didn't really want us gone.

It would have probably been smarter to just gather our immediate belongings, walk out the front door and keep on going, but Otis had ambitions to clean everything up right, to pack each piece of Mystery Junk in sturdy boxes. The process was interminable and Cleo and he functioned in an amazingly effective way. They were almost partners. Like good spouses. Then he came upon a packing dilemma he couldn't really handle.

"Mama, what about Bo?" I was standing in the kitchen next to Cleo and I saw the "not now" look she gave him. Hold on there, my Lady. We do not have secrets from *me*. You only *think* you've seen my worst anxiety attack. She accepted my pleas, and soon, as always, I was learning more than I ever wanted to know.

The only "Bo" I'd heard of was their beloved dog who died before I was born. A Boston terrier ("the smartest animal in the entire world") who lived for more than fifteen years ("he was in perfect shape – an example of the ideal athlete."). All the things they'd said about him over the years were really kinda normal. Dog lovers overrate their pets and the antics, the abilities, the affection all take on mythic proportions. It was one area in their lives that sounded right, and I liked the canine stories for exactly that reason. But oh, the memory of dear Bo was not destined to remain anyone's object of normalcy.

"What about Bo?" There was no immediate answer. It was silent for a full minute. I thought perhaps the world had ended.

"Well, honey, I just don't know..." the woman who said that looked exactly like Cleo. But who was she, this person who admitted not knowing what to do?

"I guess I'll have to." One of them said.

"Yeah. I guess maybe we do now." Some voice spoke.

"Why did this happen? Why are they making us leave?" Doesn't matter who said it. What's important is that we were back to rambling, and the earth turned again. Otis went off to the bathroom and stayed in there for a very long time. He had a lot to do.

It seems that nineteen years ago, the love of their lives (before me, of course) passed away of natural causes after *a long and wonderful life.* Cleo used to believe that one day soon they'd be able to move to a house with a yard. Maybe even *buy* something and stop losing all that monthly rent down the drain. Otis dreamed of moving out to the country. Peace and quiet. No shades to tape shut. Mary Jane hoped they could move close to someplace exciting, someplace bustling. They might live in the suburbs maybe a train-ride away from the big city. Everyone had dreams as people always do. "a place where we could bury our poor Bo..." Cleo said, actually trying to make her explanation sound sensible. "We could bury him under a big tree if we had a back yard..."

The short of it is this:

- They believed a house with a yard loomed in their future.
- They wanted Bo with them.
- He died.
- So they needed to hang onto the body .

Lacking a good plot of ground, Otis wrapped Bo in a sheet "real secure, nice and air-tight like the Egyptians did." Then another sheet (for lining). Then a towel (for softness). Then a box. But that good clump of earth was still painfully lacking. The bathroom wall hamper would have to suffice. No one expected that much time to go by. Cleo could only offer "You know how it is, when day just turns into day." We had a basement! Why on earth would you put him in the bathroom?! "Oh, honey, I don't know. Downstairs was so dirty and awful....and we didn't know what was down there..."

So for twenty-one years, Bo–the-dead-dog lay in the bottom of the corner hamper next to the bathtub. Otis pounded long nails into the hamper door, twisting them around the sides so absolutely no one could open it without literally ripping the door off its hinges. Nine-inch black nails to keep a plywood door shut, but it never seemed strange. "Oh, it's messy there, honey..." Cleo said once when I touched it. "And that door could swing open and hit me on the leg. We'd rather leave it closed." And that was that. When the fateful day came and a decision had to be made, Otis swears he opened up his carefully swaddled package to discover that Bo was still in tact. "Just like a mummy" The man who believed in no. god bowed his head. But within a matter of seconds, it seems, doggie had disintegrated to dust, the image of

Bo's perfectly preserved outline sifting through itself until there was nothing left but air. "It was really something to see..." Otis would be sharing beer that night.

After his story was told and told again, after Cleo had smiled with tears in her eyes, after Mary Jane had kissed her framed photographs of the departed Bozo, well, after all that there just wasn't anything left to be said. The dog was gone, and literally this time. Blown into the earth's wind, no longer in his homemade casket. So they justified for a while. Then they simply pitched the old box, saying the important thing was that he would always be with them in spirit.

It was clear they all three realized it was more than odd, keeping him for nearly two decades. But what day would they have decided differently? On what exact day on a calendar could they have said "okay, we're not going to get a big house with a yard...better reconsider that corpse in our bathroom..." At what precise moment should they have noticed how much time had gone by, and summoned up the courage to face just how long they'd been keeping pipe dreams going?

Enshrined in his cardboard tomb, Bo represented a better day to come. A macabre choice that may have been less about death than of *living*.

"You were a teenager and she was still going into the bathroom with you?" Yep. I know. I was a disgusting child. "What made her finally stop?" Well, now, that is another story, ain't it?

I lived in my head as a kid. I've already told you that, so nothing should be much of a shock. I had fantasies, sexual fantasies from the time I was in grade school. The Latency Period drove right past our house.

I'd pick movie stars (doesn't that go without saying?) and pretend things in my head. One man, one woman, and I was directing the inner film. Yeah, isn't that cute how she had little romances in her mind?

"Why are you so bitter about yourself?"

"I'm a realist."

"Since when?"   You just can't put a price on this kind of help.

The other day in that room with you...I don't know. I dunno. Home tonight and alone. At ease. Sometimes it's been known to happen. Anyway, you were asking me what made Cleo finally stop, and I think you're expecting some trauma drama when in fact, it's not a big deal at all. It's just that I the consummate game player couldn't give you a straight answer. I will tell ya, of course, I will. But what must it be like for you, sitting there day after day with me? Hell, you might as well be perched on the edge of the tub. When other people have trouble telling things, I figure its because they're afraid. Not humiliated. It's not because most of them are so fucking ashamed. Fear is so much classier.

Connor. I've imagined her for so long that I have no idea how she started. And don't care. I used to pretend she lived in an orphanage and detested everyone around her. She was a teenager, beautiful and wild. Disturbed a little, well maybe a lot. She ended up in a mental hospital, and she cut herself up, used to slice into her own flesh. The doctors hated her, resented her, and there was usually one in particular with whom she had some on-going battle. They tried to control her, there was fighting.

Violence. Sexual favors. She acted as a whore sometimes just to get her way. Dominance games of all sorts. I was a disgusting child.

"So ya had a very active fantasy life..." You still love to wrap everything in Velveeta cheese and make a nice table.

Anyway, that's sex for me, okay? I masturbate, I fantasize, and I like the way it's set up.

"You still have thoughts about Connor, now I mean? These days?" Oh, yeah. More than ever.

It makes no sense that I'm bringing you into all this. But what's gotten a little out of control lately is that I find myself trying to say things like her, and act like her when I'm here with you. I'm using you the way the men used me at Lara's. You charge a bit more though, for *your* fifty-minute hour.

"That can certainly be a part of what happens in treatment – playing out all kinds of fantasies…"

Non-pulsed. It's kinda cute.

"I want it to stop though. That's why I brought it up. It's a waste of both our time."

"I don't think so." Such a serious face. "It can be *useful* to understand more about those thoughts…"

"I do understand them," the Exclusion Game. "It's just not worth going into."

"And with that, I'm dismissed."

Whose words are whose? And who's been putting them into whose mouth?

There are days when I only sit there. Trying, wanting to talk with you, wanting to feel understood. But sometimes I need help with it. When I'm just sitting there, I surely don't need you to do the same.

"I don't know… I need talk, but I don't know today. Never mind, I guess.."

Silence. You're listening, I know that. But there is nothing to say. I can't connect right now. I want to, but you seem to be going farther and farther away.

"I'm right here with you." Yeah. I do know, I guess. "What are ya thinking?" I don't know. Just trying. I'm sorry. "When you need me the most…that's when you push me away the hardest…"

Just like Connor.

I've found the ultimate way to hide from this treatment. The things I say to you now are nothing but lines Connor slams at Jack. And in the absence of any relating is only role play. You say this. And I'll be her and you be him. And let's play. Okay?

Whose words? Which mouth?

88

What on earth would you think if you ever knew this is just a game to me? That everything from my tears to my cuts are props from Jack and Connor thoughts. And you're being used as a player in a scene you don't even understand....

I remember my childhood clearly. Always have. But it doesn't seem to help.

Could be that some situations are best called 'hopeless.'

"I admit you've got an excellent memory – but your insistence that you never hide from yourself – that's not true. I think you have *partial* memories – you know the facts of what happened, but you don't have emotional connection to them. You devised a way of getting rid of your stronger feelings by giving them to a fantasy character – to someone you call "not me." And it's those things you don't fully remember that get played out in your life, again and again. That's what I mean about dissociation. Those strong feelings need to be integrated into yourself as *part* of yourself...that may be a bit too abstract ... I'll try to find another way to say it..." I understand the words, but I'm scared. What you don't realize is that I never intended to actually *do* this. Not with you, not with anyone.

"I feel like if we keep going like this...how do I know I won't fall apart? Feel worse, regress."

"You could for awhile. We can't know that. I'm not going to tell you everything will be just fine. But I *don't* think you're hopeless. *Okay?*"

There are some people who are different. And on them, techniques can be dangerous. I've always been the kind of person... I don't know. I don't. I DON'T KNOW.

Otis used to have an old car, really old. This 1952 Chevy was the closest relationship he'd ever formed outside of the family. He knew its every ping, and could "tell" with an animal instinct when the radiator was getting dry. Once a year, he'd realign the points and do a brake check. He took it a shop one summer when he had a little money, and asked them what it would cost to rebuild the carburetor. But when they suggested an overhaul of the entire transmission, he turned on his heels and drove away. It wasn't the expense, he explained. He'd be glad to put good money into that Chevy. But those mechanics didn't understand what they were saying. This was the kind of car that ran best on its own. Sometimes an owner knows. Going under the hood to tinker with anything as major as the transmission or violating the   cooling system...well, that can change a car in *fundamental* ways and not always for the better. They meant well, he said, but they don't understand this Chevy. It knows how to run best on its own.

It's started up again. The cutting. I sit and stare at five slashes on my forearm. Long sleeves for work. Gotta. I kept thinking about doing it, should I? Would I? Until it just became more efficient to pick up the blade and get it over with.

"We do have to talk about this," Strauss says first thing. "It's serious..."

"I was so fed up the other day at the office," I start. Well, I had to tell him. It wouldn't feel right to keep this secret. "Elaine was pushing me, trying to get me to go somewhere with her...she's nice, and I liked her, but she's wanting too much lately..." And I knew you wanted me to go off with her, be her friend, to do whatever she asked. Just be with *her*, and leave you alone. "I don't like having to tell you this..." I only made a couple of tiny slits in my own skin. Not the end of the world.

"What is it exactly that you don't like having to tell me?" *This* – the cutting. What I did, what I do. "How scary it must be to have to do that to yourself – to not have words to say how you're feeling."

The truth is, honey, it's not the least bit scary. I'll wallow a bit in the sympathy since that's not the easiest thing to get from you these days, but your concern is misplaced. I know what I'm doing when I cut. It's not like I'm taken over by something. I'm angry. I'm feeling too much. I slice. Not the big deal all the books make it out to be. Not nearly as bad as other things I do. Things inside, that don't show blood. But, oh, that cutting is serious business. All the uproar must have to do with insurance.

"Can I see?" He asks but doesn't move. "Your arm? Can I see where you cut it?" I knew that was coming, of course. The "doctor" part of your name means you need to be sure it's not infected or dangerously bad. Just checking, right?

Sliding up my sleeve and hating it. Embarrassing to view it through your eyes. See, not so deep. Relax.

"Last week we were talking about sexual feelings. Then today you come in here and show me your body. But not in a pleasing way. Think about that one some more." And right before the session ends. "One more thing. I disagree with you. Strongly. I think you walked in here today wanting very *much* to tell me all about it."

Are you such a fucking saint that you can't admit even to yourself how much you despise me?

Cleo liked buying me jewelry, especially gold and silver chains. They weren't real of course, but they weren't cheap either. She saved a little here and a bit more there, and without anyone noticing we were on a budget, suddenly she had a wad of cash for every holiday. One of the better downtown department stores was called D. H. Holmes (as a kid I thought it must be spelled h-o-m-e, for who in this world wouldn't want to live there?). We spent countless Saturdays wandering the aisles, detouring ourselves. Nothing bad could ever happen there, that was clear. Dusty pink walls, soft track lights, an atmosphere that seemed to bless people who came through. Customers calm and dignified. Beauty as safety.

There were necklaces hanging from a velvet rope and we touched and tried them, and finally she bought me one as a surprise. A delicate string of gold links for my own body, a piece of Holmes taken into me. I loved to reach up and feel it around my neck; it was a coolness I could almost taste. Icicles draping across my chest, refined, gentle. Barely touching at all. Hints of something rather than the ever-present "too much." And as birthdays and Christmases came, she offered more chains, more delicacies and I loved her for seeing how much they mattered. Loved her for seeing me.

91

Dozens of chains in a jewelry box can get horribly tangled. Sometimes I'd reach for one, but pick up several.. It seemed that all they had to do was merely touch one another to intertwine, and such untangling of a magician's rings couldn't be done in a hurry. I'd get to it in the quiet of evening when I was fairly calm, and carefully start turning them in my fingers, at first seeing if they'd untangle by themselves if jostled. The more persistent clumps had to be teased apart with a needle, a lift here, a slide there, following the links, rolling knots. Too fast and the whole thing could get worse, too slow and one lost the thread.

"Most of the real work," Strauss says "gets done in periods of relative tranquility. We can't really sort through things while we're putting out brush fires." Wrapped tight as a strand of DNA, coiled around itself, sometimes trapped within its own links. The harder knots, ones overlapping with other chains need to separate slowly, a piece at a time. Raised up, looking good there, slowly, careful...because one link's freedom could tighten the remaining knot. Caution. The saddest thing is to get angry and pull till it breaks.

Yes, I *did* want to tell you about the cutting. And even more on target when you asked exactly what part I dreaded telling. The secret there, behind the blood line, is that I felt you were pushing me off on Elaine, telling me to form new friendships. Telling me to get away from you. And I cut. Out of pure rage.

"At me," he offers. "That knife was aimed at me." That's too easy. Too obvious. "Or too true." I didn't want to hurt you. It was about you, maybe. Yes, okay it was....but not an assault against you. I wanted you to see ME - remember me, here? "You were blaming me for all the feelings you've had lately, and ya wanted to show me how painful they are..." Well, Cleo acted like it never happened! I cut myself sometimes and she had to see it, she had to! And she pretended it was accidental. Like I didn't really do it, or have the right... Strauss listens, unconvinced. "I do think this last experience was about *us*, though. About how you're feeling towards *me*."

I'm not so good at talking directly about anything. Instead, let's dress things up a bit, a nice little outfit that makes it look like something else. A bunny suit for Easter, or a snappy elf-hat on St. Nick's Day. Let's not call any spades by nasty names here.

It's too rough on people to make them hear things undisguised. I'm sparing you as I talk again about what my family did - how I suffered long and hard so many years ago, and if you happen to see any parallels to now, well so be it. No pressure. Yes, I prefer my communiqués coded, please. Dash, dot, dot. Dot. Dash dash dash. Decipher privately, face what you can handle and ignore the rest.

"We can name things here," he insists. "And say they're about what they're really about. It won't hurt us, this relationship. We'll survive it."

You wouldn't say that if you knew.

"Then try me. Test it..." he laughs. "Ya sure test me in *other* ways!" What the hell are you talking about? Silence. The clock isn't even nearby. No watch, no time. "What are ya thinkin'?" Without word or warning, tears that I fight to keep inside my eyes. "Did that hurt your feelings..."

"No. Something else. Just thinking..."

"I wasn't angry," he says gently. "That's part of what happens here, trying things out, testing things, testing me..." I know. I understand. But I don't do things like that. "Don't go away in your head. It doesn't serve you..." Then help me! HELP ME!

"I can't feel you..." My hands look strange, not mine, not anyone's...

"I'm right here." I know. It's not a visual deficiency. The hour's almost up. I keep my eyes on the clock, letting him know that I see. "Tell me what's going on now..."

"The hour's almost up."

"It's okay. You can tell me..."

Like this, I guess. The testing. I push our boundaries. Limits.

Prove that you care by letting me slide right into the next patient's time.

"How *can* you stand me?" It is one goddamn sincere question.

"For being human?"

This is not how I came in here. I presented myself a different way, and you knock down walls and we find the cracks and one day, you're stuck with what I really am. And that is not who you agreed to see.

"I would despise me..."

"For testing me?"

"For tricking you."

"Ya really haven't. That's the bad news. The only person you fool is yourself..."

"Connor is *part* of you. You've spent a lot of energy trying not to see that..." Well, I sure see it now, brother.

Every pair of jeans I own now have cuts and shreds and dangling frays, and it's starting to extend to other items of day wear. Casey honestly seems to believe I've finally gone insane. It's a diagnosis she's based mostly on fashion, and I catch her staring at the cuts in my clothes as if they were bleeding. At first, in her inimitable style, she tried to critique my rips, offering suggestions about where exactly to cut based on pictures in Vogue and Harper's. It ain't haut couture, babe, and I couldn't care less about if I'm doing it "right." Strauss knows better than to comment and has quietly been enjoying the show. Every session some new piece of black rayon or silk slides somewhere, and fabric around my stomach is shredded and soft. A large cut along the side of one thigh – in the jeans, not the flesh. The skin stays smooth, unhurt these days. Creamy, untouched. I fondle scraggly threads above my knee. When I'm upset I yank them, twisting hard. Mostly I stroke them, petting the frays, texture between fingers. And I always wonder if he's watching.

We're less than six feet from each other.

But let us not forget, please, I am a little mad.

At Lara's I spent every day trying to seduce and arouse. Trying whatever might work, what all might please. And never once in those moments was I aware of myself at all. I was a give-away, window dressing for the task at hand. Numb to any shame or heat. See me, kiss me, pay me, bye. Flesh by Plastic Works.

But on Mondays and Thursdays in that session room, with only a single rip on one thigh, I feel totally naked. Aware of being a body. Of me in my own skin. This is madness.

Casey and I spend the evening with her long-time buddy Hal who's just finished an EST-ian weekend and emerged looking for new fish to enroll. He rambles about transformation, the realizing of one's potential and Casey, this brilliant talented woman sits at his feet, enraptured. Hal is even gay, so it can't be her usual loss of intellect that results from romantic love. She later swears that what he described is a combination of eastern metaphysics and the best of behavioral therapies. Yes, I "get it." You plan to do the Enlightenment Weekend. A year ago, I wouldn't have considered letting her do such a thing without me. No one should evolve alone, as that could result in distancing from the "untransformed" people in one's life. So, I would have sat right there with her. Hell, I would have paid for us both. I would have been her Cleo and whenever she looked into my face, she would see nothing but approval. I can't do it anymore. Well, doctor, you've now taken away the only remaining thing I ever cared about.

"Hal really likes you," she offers later. He must need *two* people to sign up. Okay, a bit harsh. One night when she was out, he called me with questions about some recipe (as if) and we chatted for an hour. Once again, he'd just broken up with Mr. Wrong, and since Casey wasn't around, he accepted solace from whoever answered the hot line. He's not a bad guy. He's not. He's just a would-be actor with no money and a lousy job and he picks awful partners and he talks too much and he has no absolutely no sense of how he comes across. And like everyone, he takes too much energy. "He said you were so insightful." He likes a shiny mirror, I guess. Most folks do.

The next day he calls again, still trying to sell me on joining Casey for the experience of our lives, adding that if I'm short of cash, he can offer a loan. One cannot let money stand in the way of learning our true potentials. It seems this is the dawning of a new era in humanity's history. We are to lead the others, we the enlightened, and the self-awareness that we create our own realities will spread like wildfire throughout the world. A thought is a thing, an energy force. What we humans believe and live by is the very reality we manifest in concrete form. In short, we're god, and that's the Secret of the ages that has been withheld. How could I turn down a chance to alter the world?

Hoping I'll change my mind soon, he blesses me, releases me and lets me go. This is a guy who can't get one thing in his mortal life to work, but now he's ready to try his hand at being the Almighty. And I'm the one on Stellazine.

That part of me, glib and observant – it's like I have a Reporter-person hiding in my brain. I *can* see what's normal, what's odd, what's comical...but it's only one way of looking. This CNN anchorwoman who sees and analyzes, she herself is a defense, a technique to cope - because beneath her sensible eyes, there's still Me. Me who again and again with oblivion to all parlor wit, is still sick, as sick and confused as if I couldn't tell what was sensible at all. A secret is that I envy people who can't fake it. The delirious madwoman who claws and raves. At least it's real, such raw energy and bleak terror upon whose face no mask can fit. Such people get to live full out as they feel. Yes, its hell. It's genuine. And yes, I'm bitter. The people I pretend for, they can't even see. NO one can tell what I've gone through in an effort to stay out here in this world. That's becoming clearer at least. No one at all understands.

Mid-way through session. (at least I get upset earlier in the hour lately)

"I...because I'm not myself around anybody..."

"And that's their fault?"

Why can't you help me find something good to do for a living? Get me out of that job, help me to write or perform more...why can't we focus on that?"

"If you want to talk about those things, we can. I only follow your lead." That is such crap. "And if you have an *opinion* about what I just said – not reading your mind, I can read your face!...tell me so. Don't go off in your head. Devalue me *out here*."

"I don't understand what it is you want from me."

"There we go again." I know. I know. I'm sorry.

YOU DO NOT KNOW ME.

I still nurture the hope that out there somewhere lies the perfect mental hospital for me when that time inevitably comes. It will be majestic and white, a Magic Mountain-type facility where I can finally rest and be cared for. It's a place where no one talks loudly and gentle hands offer soothing pills as ethereal patients nod to one another, strolling across plush gardens. That is, however, not the institution where my mother landed.

Mary Jane's special little rest took place in Charity Hospital, what with our recurring issue of poverty. She went to heal in a place where no human being could even exhale, where screams and sobs of attention-seeking misery blew through the night, and shuffling feet bumped into her in the halls. Clearly, it offered less of a rest than a *warning*, and in that fashion, such a visit can be effective. *See what happens to those who can't hide it? This is the final stop for people who insist on being seen for who they are. Want to rethink it now? Like another shot out in the world? Maybe next time you'll fasten your mask on a little tighter.*

Cleo had tried every resource not to send her. ("The worst thing I ever did in my life...") But when Mary Jane didn't sleep for six nights, and her incessant talking grew louder by the hour, there was no place to go but away. By Day 7 her voice was so hoarse that it sounded like a man, and her words strange and frantic sounded like she was channeling a demon. Small wonder that in Days of Old, psychotics were labeled "possessed" and in lieu of Haldol, an exorcism was shoved down their throats.

And as always, I report the facts, that's all, sounding as if I had a grip. I sound. My mind was breaking apart, but I at that moment I stood second to the real Madwoman. Cleo needed me to not to need. To appear okay. I held the world together with my lies.

As her talking got louder (always perfectly timed to the darkest moment in the middle of the night) Cleo took her into the bathroom because "sounds are insulated better in there." By the time Day Two of porcelain living rolled around, Otis had devised a plan. Since the upstairs neighbors were the potential problem, and since it was through their floor that yelling needed to be muffled...anyway, the result was Otis on a ladder with six towels, five old comforters and lots of duct tape. Carefully adhered to Mary Jane's bedroom ceiling, the soft insulation could work wonders. He talked about a trip to the Salvation Army the next day so he could buy fluff in bulk and fasten it to all four surrounding walls. Yep, Otis was prepared to construct the one thing we'd been missing – a padded room. Sadly, it wasn't meant to be. I know how those poor carpenters can sling blame, but sometimes it's true. Cleo refused to let him use nails on his insulation ("honey, that could be almost more disturbing that the hollering...") and duct tape is after all, guaranteed to be *very* strong. "He's a genius!" Cleo cried when she saw his puffy Sistine masterpiece where he'd even tried to match patterns and color. Pink flowers touched green solids and were far away from orange stripes.

It was remarkably weird, but it really might've worked - if not for that unfortunately heavy brown comforter that slowly pulled its way free from the tape. If only it hadn't picked the exact moment to drop from the ceiling just as Mary Jane entered her new sanctuary, things could have been okay. But even for someone *not* in a psychotic state of confusion, it can be pretty scary to have (apparently from nowhere) a giant blanket land on your head. Shrieks and tears and cries about traps and police and lights, so many lights all over the neighborhood to shine a path for the ambulance.

Nine hours later Cleo came back in a taxi. All she said was how awful the place was, and that it was wrong to have Mary Jane there. Within three days, my mother was home. Those three days are gone from my memory, but when Cleo got out of the cab that morning, she wasn't her. Eyes hold the soul and her soul always adored me. Her heart was my heart, her hands on my arms or from my arms, extensions of me. Our body. But when she came home, she was not her. Cleo was not the one who was crazy, she was not the one in the hospital. Nothing should have happened like it did. Nothing should have changed.

"Some say the world will end in fire..."

I stand with those who favor ice. I know what kills.

A month later I was in some psychiatrist's office heeding words from the Good Book of St. Cleo. "Only tell him what you *have* to so you can get more valium." And Elavil. Maybe a bit of Mellaril if those don't work out. School was no longer an option.

"Tell me more about that – when your grandmother turned to ice..."

It didn't happen often, really. It was okay, but there were times, sometimes that day and after when she stopped being her. Some people get angry and they show it, right? *You* do - I can tell when you're annoyed. But Cleo never gave me anything but eyes of admiration. Well, *adoration*, to say it right. Except sometimes at those times, it was never her fault but when things overwhelmed her, the only way out for her was...out."

She looked at me with nothingness. I could always get her to come back, she and I had this bond, of course. And I'd work to charm for hours at a time, and then finally she returned into her own eyes...and mine.

On or off. Masked or headless. Heat or ice.

People all take so much energy, but nobody wants to hear.

What did you say to upset Mary Jane?
The question should be carved into my tombstone.

I once tried to joke with her, that woman, my mother. I was only teasing and I wasn't mean. Let us please know that I have meanness in me - I have *hatred* in me, but I am not completely insane and I know if I'm being mean.

Teasing is sexual. Do most children know? I feel it in my crotch and I understand games and I don't play by rules unless I respect you. I tried to flirt with her once, that woman, my mother. Verbally playful, well I used to be. Telling jokes in Freud's mind is filled with aggression, and the assault of forcing someone to laugh is a rape of friendly proportions. I cannot help that I'm funny.

The saddest fact of schizophrenia is not the delusions or paranoia. Its cruelest symptom may be that every joke becomes a rapier sword. It's an illness that turns laughter into pain.

We sit on the bed, she and I, I and she. And she studies me, as always. Looking for the inanimate doll she wishes for, so pretty, so sweet, so still. Dead as porcelain, obedient as the pin-up of Lana. Posed. Threatless. Cool as paper. I was "such a good girl," they always said, and it just isn't true. I cried and whined and demanded my own way. But when the need arose, there was no one more compliant. I did whatever Cleo needed and in exchange, she was mine.

There comes a point in every sado-masochistic waltz when the lights go on, and the truth is out. *I am completely your slave now, through and through. There is nothing I would ever refuse you. So for my next trick, let me tilt the world. And north is south, and you are my object. Who owns who now, babe? Get it?*

Wednesday. Noon. (extra session)

"I can't stand my job anymore. It's unbearable..." He lets me whimper but refuses to toss my lips any fish. Help me. Goddamn you in fucking heaven, help me! "I know you think I'm being such a baby, but it's literally torture being there. You can't know. I'm sorry, but you just can't, because you don't totally understand. I'm so much sicker than anyone realizes."

"If I didn't hear this with my own ears, every single session, I wouldn't believe it. Not a day goes by without you telling me that I have no idea how bad off you really are."

"I'm sorry..."

"Let's look at *that*, too, your apology – as if you've done something bad. "

"Okay, you're right. Apologizing is just a reflex."

" Maybe *not*. Maybe you're aware of what's *behind* your words every time you insist I don't understand. And that's why you feel the need to be sorry." I'm just being polite, that's all. I

100

was trying... "See, I think it's very *aggressive* when you tell me that." And he watches my face for an appraisal as to how that may have landed. It's my clue that he thinks he's said something crucial. "It's the worst indictment you could make of me as a caretaker – that I'm not empathic." His face is one of the few I can look at these days. Please don't be angry. "It's *hostile*, right? Can ya see that?" A nod, eyes not leaving me. "And you insist on holding onto believing it - convinced you're misunderstood is a way of saying 'fuck you."

"Okay, okay." Chill. Breathe. He doesn't look mad, but I never know. I'm sorry, I'm sorry, I'm sorry – no, wait, that's what got us *into* all this. There really aren't words. For anything. "What about the old promise that a person can say *whatever they want* in therapy, be any way, and what's the phrase... you'll provide "unconditional positive regard?"

"Oh, no, I *never* said *that!*" Eyes smiling, not needing caution at all.

"Cleo, can you come play?" Well, hell's bells, guys...all children have urges.

"So Casey's having more problems?" I swear the doctor looks bored.

"Alan really let her down..." I've been up all night talking with her, trying to find answers. Unable to find someone good to love, she herself is breaking. This dear wonderful woman, lost to herself sometimes, just picks the wrong men, tries to see someone who isn't there.

"She sets herself up to be hurt," Yes, I see that. Of course I see it. But she *can't*, and it's too cruel to shove that down her throat.

"Is it?" He asks so seriously. "Or is it more cruel to keep playing along?"

Cleo's face would shine every time any of us entered the room. Shouldn't that alone have been enough to keep us all sane?

I listen to the words of people who had terrible childhoods, told they were unwanted, resented, even despised. And those words always end with their conviction that they're troubled today because they weren't loved. May be true. Then how can anyone explain me?

"It has to be biological," I keep pleading. And responding in kind, he offers the latest meds. A Xanax or Valium is crucial these days. Wouldn't be leaving the house without 'em. The newer anti-depressants help, but they almost seem to be soothing a part I didn't even know was hurt. But the major fears, those stay untouched.

"How do they help? Can you describe it?"

" Maybe they make me not hate so much."

"Not hate your*self*," he adds. But I keep reading of people whose lives are transformed with the perfect prescription. Why not me... Why never me. ..

"I wish we could find the right medicine..." I'm feeling bold. "Or maybe there isn't any."

"No magic pills, no. And with you, with what goes on in your mind, those awful states you get into - it's not caused from something bio-chemical..."

"I am not doing this to myself!"

He looks like he has no idea where to go next. I shouldn't have settled on such a nice guy for a doctor. A real bastard would at least deserve me.

"Is that what you honestly think?" I ask a week later. "That I do this to myself?!"

"You want to fight with me..."

"Actually I want you to *agree* with me, but hey, if not, then fighting is an option..."

"Why does it matter if I agree with you?"

"Why does it matter to *you* if *I* do?"

"*You* are the one in treatment here..." I don't even want to fight today, but it's where I go. It's the only place I feel safe with you.

Casey's heart isn't healing, and slowly the "cancer" has spread to Late Notices, rent-paying, borrowers and lenders be...her finances have reached an irreparable uproar. This child-woman is like so many in New York, recognizable on buses and in restaurants as they cry to a sympathetic friend and lick up words like saucer-milk, all they need are words that reassure. *"you deserve more...how could he?...it'll get better...your time is due...you don't feel entitled to take care of yourself... you're a trusting person who gives too much...."*

But these women would gasp and turn white if they heard of a person such as me who takes sharp objects and slices neat marks deep into her own skin, who sometimes can't feel anything at all without a little blood appearing, and sneaks peaks beneath her perennial long-sleeves to find macabre comfort in watching the progress of her self-inflicted wounds. How sick. How...crazy. How sad. I know. But what the Caseys of this world don't know is that they use sharp objects, too. They slice up their own hearts and lives and careers and hopes. Instead of knives or razors, they use men and credit cards and have no idea that they're self-inflictors.

"You're absolutely right," This can't be *Strauss* saying such a thing. "You see what she *can't* – that *she's* doing this – to herself..." Then a long stare, like you're *willing* something into me. Man, chill. That look could drive a real psychotic into the land of No Return.

Anyway, I see what you want me to see. Fuck you. I get it.

"...and what I try to point out, is that you also..."

"I get it." If you're right, just if....how do I stop?

With that two-step forward, I need to race back one long big one. Home from work early, and by 4:00, I'm way deep into the Crazy Thing. It's *choice* (happy, Strauss?). At least at first, it is. By nightfall I'm a mere passenger.

"You hide in acting crazy..." Yes. You're right. Sometimes I do. I play many, many games, see. Every morning that I show up for work is one more Meryl Streep-quality performance. Every time I sit in a restaurant with someone and talk and laugh when the unreality is sweeping across my skin, yes, I hide in playing like I'm all right. But those kinds of roles don't last. I step off the stage and those games end. But the Crazy thing, ah that takes me aaalllll the way home....

Madness is time gone haywire. This afternoon I stood by the copier and it seemed like Time itself had made a quantum leap. I was actually at home perhaps, and suddenly in a quirk of chaos, I appeared at work...but part of me was still back there...like a ghost-image from a poorly adjusted TV, a trail of Self wafts off the body, a wisp of soul quivers away. I'm dying, or worse. Vanishing into nothingness and forced to stay conscious to witness it all. I need someone to adjust the controls and pack me back in, back into my body, my mind...I'm drifting, shadows of soul lost in the Xerox room, trails of me left like breadcrumbs on the hall floors of the firm...and when I get to the street, I'll be nothing but twigs. Bones baked hard in a crematorium that fly like soot through the streets of the city. ("Needing to go home. Migraine pretty bad.") Racing to my door to recapture the part of me that didn't leave in time, that couldn't catch up to the rest of me ... retracing steps, rekindled selves. God help me. Don't tell me I'm not mad.

"It hasn't been that bad in a long time, right?" Right. Let's take that much at least.

My neighbor seen in the elevator did not look like himself. No one does lately. Like the soap operas Cleo and I used to watch. If one of the regular actors got sick, there was a voiceover at the beginning of the show providing a little clarity. "Today the role of Miranda will be played by Stacy Bennett..." And then an unknown face appeared in Miranda's clothes, and proceeded to kiss Miranda's men and everyone pretended nothing was strange. If you'd just tuned in, if you weren't a regular fan, you'd never know it wasn't her.

Cleo looks at me, but there is no voice to tell me who she is today.

It's started with Casey now. The mirror did it, no, Cleo I know the mirror didn't really do anything (I'm trying hard, my love, not to sound too nuts). Casey was putting on make-up in the bathroom and when I stood behind her and glanced at her reflection, her face was different. Yes, for crying out loud, I know we all look peculiar mirror-imaged. It was more than that. Someone else is showing up in her clothes, in her stead. I know better. I do. I do know better than that. The knowing just doesn't help.

"You're seeing something different in her lately," he offers and then sees my face. "Although I can tell you're not interested in going down that path..."

"I just..." how to ask you. To beg you not to talk down to me. "Can I say something without *you* getting defensive?"

"With that introduction, probably not." He chuckles. "But say it anyway. I can take it."

'You're very intelligent," I start.

"So far, I'm not defensive at *all*...."

"Yeah, well, be patient."

"Oh, I am *nothing* if not patient..." Okay now, there's enough here for twenty sessions (ten for each of us). I know what he means, of course. I *know* this is not the swiftest of treatments. Then *listen* to me, I want to say. If there's no time to spare, cut the wisecracks.

It's not true though, that we can't afford the time to play. Years ago, I interviewed a therapist who asked me three times in our first (and only) session why I felt the need to make little jokes. He insisted I did not have to be funny, on and on... I wanted to say, *maybe I'm not trying to entertain **you**, jack ass.* A little amusement keeps *me* going. Mostly I hated that he called them "little jokes." Lacking a similar wit, we didn't stand a prayer of connecting through my pain.

Dr. Strauss must have a few children patients, and on one bookcase stands a game box of Candyland, some coloring books, jacks and a ball. Less toys, more necessary tools of the trade. I saw a drawing up there last week that bore the name "Alicia." She probably gave it to him when the session was over, leaving behind a piece of herself. He couldn't have gotten Alicia to talk very much if he just sat there in his chair, smiled and waited. She wouldn't have believed him if he'd said, "you can tell me what's wrong, honey...and I'll help you." Must have been so scared, poor kid, going to see this doctor who promised not to hurt.

He had to earn her trust. She needed to see how he plays. How he wins, how he loses. If he cheats, and how he acts when one of them gets caught. And to know he was watching for the same in her.

I couldn't have made it this far without the toys.

Cleo, my wonderful love, always wanted us to be romantic and poignant and dear. No room for combat or even warm sparks of conflict. Angry stoked up fires were only in my mind. And Connor did what I couldn't, was treated all the ways I was not. And her bad girl style was the secret fantasy I kept even from Cleo. I was adored and revered. And Connor was the anti-me.

With Cleo I was Cathy to her Heathcliff, what a beauty she is, I am, always told me how lovely I was…my hair and him…the charm, how charming he could be with her. He was kind and doting, they/we were lovers well cast. What I remember the most about playing was how loud and long we'd laugh at the end. *Aren't people so silly*??? One of us never failed to say it, a mantra, a good luck phrase, a prayer. *Sex runs them, some people live their lives with sex running them*! The word was always run. We talked on and on about the characters we played and then about some real people we may have seen on the street…and we laughed at them with all our body and soul. Oh, how we laughed. On those nights we were wed.

I keep remembering the Strauss Theory that I'm seeing something "different" in Casey when she looks like someone else. Maybe I'm seeing more of what is there. The most extraordinary relationship of my life, that's what Casey is/was/shall be destined for… It's not acceptable that in truth, it's not so different from all others I've already had. Gametime? *I'll be Cleo and you be you…and here honey, I'll wipe you in our bathroom. I don't mind, really. I'd do anything for you.*

There's going to be a Secret Santa thing at work. I despise secrets.

Who else in the halls of our pretty little Firm is like me? I watch faces in the cafeteria, all those panty-hosed, silk-tied bodies, and it's just not possible every one is what they appear to be. Who's the secret cutter, the overeater? Which one has ever tried to die? And the most important question, which one doesn't know what's real, has beliefs about magic and madness, lives in a world as beautiful and terrifying as a nightmare?

They care about raises and promotions and what others think and vacation homes and who is invited to what party and their hair. It is unspeakable that some people get up in the morning caring about their *hair*.

"So you feel superior to those people at work," he says. "Both superior and inferior, but either way you're comparing yourself." They're in my face. I have to do something to keep from screaming bloody murder. "I think you very much would like to conform to that stereotype you talk about. Part of you wouldn't feel at home there at all, but part of you wants to blend in, no, more than that, to lose yourself. It's an archaic fantasy...an infant who thinks she and the mother are one person, wanting to merge with her..."

"Merge with them? I despise them..."

"That's the give-away. If you weren't drawn to them, you'd just say 'they're not for me' and leave it at that. But they get so much of your energy."

"Then what's my choice? If you're right, I should just give in and try to become like them?!"

"Is that actually what you think I'm saying?" No. Okay. No. "Again, there's that arguing."

"Well, I was just following what you said..." Sort of.

"But you know that's not what I meant. See, as long as you can pretend differently, and challenge me, saying how wrong I am, how I didn't understand, all that keeps us busy." I know I look confused... "And then the session will be over. And we didn't have to do much work."

What must that experience be for a doctor? To connect to someone's truth, getting inside the cave of another person's mind and, then turning around carefully, point out a stalactite that was never before seen? In the midst of it all, I feel sad that Casey can't find someone decent. Her therapists over the years all seem so blindly supportive, reinforcing her beliefs that she's only a poor misguided child. At least they try to for awhile. She's told me a few things some have said when they eventually did get challenging, and it sounds like they held it all in for so goddamn long that they finally started attacking wildly. Then Casey simply walked away confused, calling them both wrong or downright nutty. All the books say the most important thing is "fit" between doctor and patient. I'd also add luck. The right day, the right guy. Life is a fucking crap shoot.

"If she's never in her life been able to find anyone to love who's a good fit" Strauss said once, "it's not surprising that she also can't find the right therapist."

"I happen to know you're damn good, in spite of anything else I might say…"

"So it's all me, huh?"

"No. Not all…but you are extraordinary."

"Careful there. Don't idealize me. I might not survive the fall…"

"Oh, I know you're far from perfect…"

"Okay, okay…but seriously, I'm not extraordinary either. What I am is an average therapist who tries to do a reasonably competent job." You actually mean that.

"That's not true," I had to say, "Look at *me* - it's not like I'm such a good patient! You said yourself that part of me doesn't even *want* to get better!"

"And part of you does."

"The jury's still out."

"No. Part of ya *does*. That jury may be out on whether you'll *let* yourself."

"Why would someone need that?" he asks later. "To think they were extraordinary?" Well, let's see hon, everyone I know sure *does*.

And, of course, we're just hiding the fear that underneath we're seriously flawed. The curse of the narcissist. Adore me, or else I 'm nothing. And how much of that pain was Cleo's.

But back to you, sweet doctor. I don't buy it. You admit you've got your own conflicts. Well, one of them is that – you want to be both powerful and harmless. You chose a dangerous profession where your hand is on the trigger of people's lives, and then you try to bask in how ordinary you are. Not quite. Who's the narcissist from your own past you're trying so hard not to be?

The handwritten messages on our birthday cards were always compliments in superlative.

To the best, most beautiful, most wonderful, smartest, happiest, sweetest, kindest, most fun, most thoughtful, funniest, most talented...[grand daughter] or.[daughter] or [brother] or [son] or [uncle] or [mother] or [grandmother] in the world!! All my love forever and a day, all my heart and soul forever, and all my prayers and wishes for the most happiness in the world.

My.

"It seems you got inside your mother's mind, probably when you were very very young..."

Cleo would agree. She almost seemed jealous that I could understand.

Mary Jane wouldn't come in from the front porch and it was nearly dark.

"Honey, don't you want to watch TV. with Janine? She's right here." Oh, yeah, sacrifice *me*. "Janine, please sweet thing, let's ask Mary Jane to come inside..."

Oh, I dunno. She looks pretty busy. What she's actually doing is sitting in a chair and rambling away to the air. Cleo believes she thinks someone is with her, but that's wrong. It's only thoughts that can't stay inside. That's partly why her very body won't leave the porch. Half in. Keeping herself slightly outside, on a border. Too far "out there" and everything descends; too far "inside" and she'll implode. Angrier than she's been in months, she waves her arms wildly like its self-defense.

"I NEVER never in a million years would think so, never and you know! You know know know! I watched her tits, ya had her fancy dancin' all over that floor and you got hard as an angry old stone! For god's sake in the heavens, I know that!!"

"Mary Jane, honey" Cleo is too scared. "There's nobody out here..." She knows that, sweet Cleo. Haven't you ever gotten so furious that you couldn't stop thinking what you'd say the next time you saw somebody? That's all she's doing, your daughter on her porch. And she knows it's a chance long gone, so she chews on a pacifier in a scene all by herself. We all do it. We just don't let it show.

"What brought this on?" Cleo begs. "What made her get like this all of a sudden?" I did.

We were in her room (well, that's where you want me) and she was looking through magazines and watching me too close again. It was clear what she was thinking.

"Honey, stand next to that picture of Ava Gardner...." Just leave me the fuck alone. "Oh, please honey! Just stand right there so I can see something."

"I do not look like Ava Gardner." Wouldn't ya think I'd know to keep my mouth shut? But we don't do such things in our house. We're each as stubborn as the next, each as nutty as the one before. I know you're insane and I know what to do to shut you up. But why the fuck should I? I'm tired letting *your* madness always win. "If you were a man," I asked, "would you want Ava Gardner or Lana Turner?" Come one, Mom, which one do you really want to fuck?!

"You got into competition with her, for the right to be crazy..." Yep.

More every year. I even said to her once, "Back off, Helen of Hollywood. It's time for *Cassandra's* mad scene now!"

I thought of it last night, the amazing of most amazing things. How rarely I feel so dreamy anymore. How long it's been since I had those episodes. The oddest part is that in the remembering I'm doing with Strauss, nothing's coming up that I haven't remembered before. No great repressed trauma; sadly, no satanic abuse which could explain everything and clear my name once and

110

for all. No, just ordinary stuff. Ordinary for me, anyway. Left over emotions, he'd call it. Passions from other days. Covered by outmoded defenses.

Old casings of armor for wars long ago lost.

In light of no real enemies now, just re-cast, and keep the show going.

"Yep," Strauss smiles. "Then ya can take it out on the *rest* of us." I'd like to say I'm sorry, but I know better. "You pretend your psychiatrist is your grandmother. Your mother is Casey…Of course you haven't mourned them! They're *with* you every day."

Not to be negative, but…. I wonder if the price for no depersonalization is this anger I can't seem to get rid of. You've said I've been hiding emotions. So now I'll live my life as a wild rage-filled child?

"Maybe for right now. Do ya think the way you are is so awful?"

It does seem to be the popular consensus. But personally, no. I've never felt more real in my life.

Question: What did ya do for your 40th birthday?

Answer: Wasn't sure what I was in the mood for really. So I got a tattoo.

A three -our bus ride to Woodstock. A renowned body artist, well, no ordinary schmo is gonna stick sharp objects into me. I reserve that right exclusively.

A child, a wild child, a ruffian little girl coming right through my skin, climbing out, up, holding two pieces of barbed wire in her hands. She's not out of control, she looks kind of smug. A smirking little kid with scruffy hair, a cut up t-shirt and hands above her head, proudly arriving. Coming through. Being me.

111

I've now taken mirror study to a new art form, staring at my arm for an hour last night. She's the kid Mary Jane was afraid of. The kid Cleo couldn't handle. And she's not bad, she's certainly not evil, just a little wild is all. She's human, I guess. She's Connor.

"So?" I wore a sleeveless shirt just for you. "Wanna see?"

He laughs. "Sounds like ya sure want to show me." You should see who I'm turning out to be. After all.

"She's *erupting* out of your skin...with the barbed wire, of course..." I love your expression. Not shocked. Or repelled. "She's really something. Did you sketch her and take it in?"

Worked on it for a long time. Drawn and reworked. Refined. Chosen. The first "mutilation" done totally with purpose.

"Did it hurt?" Then he makes a face. "Oh, yeah, look who I'm asking...." And we laugh. Any patient ever get a tattoo before right in the middle of treatment? As evidence of change...that's part of what this is for me. Proof. Of me.

"That's something you can take with you, right?" Yes. Yes! "An emblem to prove this was real...not a dream." You honestly do seem to understand.

Casey approaches me with great caution and chalks up the tattoo to a middle-aged effort to recapture youth. All the kids are getting body art. In some ways, I probably am about fourteen these days.

"In seems like your tattoo is not only about wanting to show yourself to other people..." he offers just as the session ends. "But also about *us*. Our relationship here. As if that's a product of the work we've done together..." Yes.

It's our creation, doctor. Our child.

"You know what I think?" Now there's a good question to ask a delusional person with paranoid tendencies. "I think

112

sometimes you don't know when you *are* being genuine. So to be safe, you claim it's all pretending."

Some nights I wish I could go to the middle of Central Park and howl at the moon.

I seem to scare Casey these and Strauss thinks I represent her darker side, feelings she tries to ignore. She, of course, says she's only trying to help. Or trying to mellow out what she doesn't understand.

I've never been anyone's Dark Moon before. I was supposed to be in this world to bring only brightness. Even if I don't want to.

Who I am now is not who I ever was. There are days when I feel possessed.

It's clear that in the hands of an even slightly lesser doctor, I could turn into a Multiple right about now. I might insist on being *called* Connor, or just waltz into my next session as scared little Sybil or haughty Eve Black. Many selves, (or veils, as you call them). Peeling away, layer after layer, until...oh, yeah. That is the key word here.

To tell you more about the fantasies I've had. The sexual ones. Sometimes you're there, you know.

"What is it about Connor you're afraid to let me see?" You walk near me on the thinnest of ice.

Oh, I have more weird stories about my family though. Let's talk about *them* today.

The tales she told to the King, you see,
were shared to keep her safe. Spared.
Stalling tactics, little more.
To keep them far apart.
Never never ever ever never to bring them into each other's arms.

Lie, why?

Category 1: Society Made Her Do It

When Mary Jane found herself pregnant oh, those many years ago, it was quite the conundrum. Cleo's husband was appalled, convinced that his poor daughter would no way, no how find the wherewithal to raise a child. Yes, there was a father, yes of course. It takes two to make a baby. We know that. But it doesn't really require a man, you see. It takes a penis.

The Celebrity Lounge, a French Quarter night club next door to one of New Orleans' oldest live theatres. When Minsky's Burlesque came to town, the show folk would pour into The Lounge for their after-performance drinks. Night after night, finally in her element, there was my mother rubbing elbows with the stars. Once, so it was said, someone asked if she was a showgirl. Mr. Minsky himself had flirted with her. But yes, we all remember. "I couldn't be a show girl though! The make you do too much you might not like."

The owner of The Celebrity Lounge liked Mary Jane. He was charming, flirtatious and a bit of a phony (well, I had to get it somewhere). They were only a brief fling, these veritable strangers. A romance of a few months, if we're to believe the Cleo-Press, of course. He wasn't a guy who liked children, didn't want responsibilities, was out of the picture. Over. Painless. Done with.

An abortion that got rid of the man, not the child.

No one looked back. However, this was the early 1950's in Louisiana. Mary Jane could *not* be allowed to have an illegitimate baby.

It would be well over twenty years before I got the actual story. All I knew growing up was that my mother and father were married for a very short time and they really weren't getting along, and he didn't want children but she did, and oh, she loved me so much, and she didn't love him, and then one day he went on a business trip and the plane crashed and that was that. At six, I knew there was something fishy about that story, but I was also positive that I didn't want to know the truth. He could have been evil, a maniac, a murderer. Something awful, I knew it was awful. Let's never talk of it. Please. They were happy to meet that request.

The real story would not prove a let down in terms of nuttiness, but there was no horror to be faced. Cleo had this boyfriend on the side, see her marriage wasn't good and there was a man who worked up at the liquor store named Mr. Clay. He'd always liked her, thought she was so pretty, and of course, she'd flirted wildly to get Otis' beer put on a tab. Mr. Clay would be the sin of Cleo's life, the one mistake against which all else would be measured. But in those days, he was only a nice fellow who would do anything she asked. And that was all she needed.

On a Saturday afternoon in the fall of '53, Mr. Clay and Mary Jane took a little ride across the river. Small towns outside New Orleans did things their own way, and if there was ever a place to get married without any legitimate identification, it was in Granville. A small ceremony, one witness (guess who?), and soon my mother was wed to a totally fictitious man by the name of Ralph Baker. Cleo had let her daughter decide what to call him, much in the way children love to name their own pets. They drove home from Granville with a marriage license. All was right with the world.

"So she married your grandmother's lover?" Yep. "But didn't take his *name*? They just made *up* a name??" Why now, *why* would you look for logic?

Category 2: Because That's Just How People Are

There's a big Catholic population in New Orleans, old French and Spanish influences, large families, gothic cathedrals. Cleo realized it was the most popular religion around her, and when in Rome...

Unfortunately, our little family lacked any church-going genes at all, and they'd supposedly been baptized in The First Christian Church so many years ago, so many lifetimes ago, and no one really knew where the heck that church was or if New Orleans even had one. Anyway, most people were Catholic, and so it was decided. No, not that we would actually *become* Catholics, just that we'd all say we were.

Some things are easy to fake, for example, sanity. But Catholicism, to an untrained, uneducated consumer will offer many surprise secrets. There is this thing called First Communion, where the little child, still young enough to be sinless, goes for her first experience of tasting the body and blood of Christ. I missed that one. Then at adolescence, there's a Confirmation Ceremony where said child reaffirms her love for the Holy Trinity. I didn't know what that was and missed it too. Needless to say, my one experience of Sunday mass was a choreographic nightmare of kneeling, standing, kneeling, reciting, hand-shaking, and evermore kneeling that smacked of the Actor's Nightmare where everyone on stage but me knows their lines on opening night.

"Yes, I'm Catholic," I know I could have said it under lie-detection and not sweated a single bullet. Kids at school asked what church we went to, but luckily I was considered odd enough that if I didn't answer, no one got suspicious.

One day I said somebody had said something about The Lord's Prayer, and when Cleo heard that, she got a little pale.

"You mean, you don't know the Lord's Prayer?" Excuse me? At what point that I am never out of your sight did you imagine I would have been taking a Religion Correspondence Course? So we sat in the kitchen and had a memorization lesson. "You have to know that one, honey, oh, you just have to..." I was so terrified of being caught with my Lord's prayer down around my knees that I repeated it for two solid hours. "Oh, you are so smart!" she praised. And it's a damn good thing, I thought, or we'd all be going to hell.

Category 3: What <u>Was</u> She Thinking?!?!
a/k/a
Come Back, Little Sofa!
Our couch is being reupholstered.

There were a couple of nice pieces of furniture in our living room, but they were very old and not well maintained. A chest of drawers and its matching end tables were souvenirs from a better time, when Cleo was first married and money was rarely an issue. Nearly a hundred porcelain figurines covered every surface, with trinkets from Woolworth's and hand-made keepsakes stacked on top of each other in huddled piles. Our lamps were too big for their shades, and there is just nothing like a nice set of plastic curtains to really finish off a room. We had too many chairs and few memories of where they'd even come from. There was hardly a path to walk without careening around an old hassock, or collector's stack of T. V. Guides. But against the wall, right beneath the window was a large empty space, six feet by three feet to be exact. No. It was not space for a coffin.

We had no couch. Simple truth. Unfortunate, yes, but in the big BIG scheme of things, not such a horrible fact. Except to Cleo. "*Everyone* has a nice couch!" she almost sounded angry at me. Okay, okay. Forget it. Okay. When anyone entered our house, and lord that was not so often, we casually mentioned that our couch was out being reupholstered. This was not necessarily the easiest thing to introduce into conversation, but we each mastered our own way of handling it. (It is so clear why I'm good at Improv.) The landlord coming in to check a bad leak didn't bat an eye when he realized that the fugitive sofa was still missing after several years. One of my (braver) school friends came over to spend the afternoon and looked positively frightened when Otis cornered her on the way to the bathroom and started explaining away the mysterious lack of couch-ness in our home. The topic even bled into Mary Jane's psychoses when she suspected that the government knew the truth about our un-sofa and were diligently keeping records of all that was said.

Once I asked Cleo what she thought the "couch" looked like, and she laughed and quickly described a dark hunter green velvet with burgundy throw pillows. I'd always pictured chintz, but hey, it wasn't *my* piece of furniture.

"So even after you started menstruating, she was still helping you in the bathroom..." Don't think it's not seen, your carefulness. If you were too explicit, especially at first, I wouldn't have been able to do this at all. Even now, you use words only if I do. Say "wiped" only if I have. For someone so blatantly sarcastic (in safer areas), you are one hell of a guy to monitor when thicker kid gloves are needed. Don't think it goes unnoticed.

Fourteen is really not *so* old. Do ya think?

Anyway, it wasn't a big deal. The day it all occurred to me. I just thought maybe I should tell her that I could do it myself, I guess. It was time, I thought, for her to not have to do that for me anymore. That's all. But I hated to tell her, couldn't find the right time. Guess a smart place to look might be while she sat on the edge of the tub one foot in front of me, but I didn't want her to think I didn't need her, or didn't appreciate it. And she never seemed to mind.

In fantasy, see, Connor just couldn't take anybody touching her at all. She wanted everyone's hands to cut it fucking out, and leave her alone and stay over there and okay, okay come in if you need to, but we don't have to touch. So I played (in my favorite spot, alone in my head) and imagined she got so worked up that she found a way to stop it once and for all.

There was an old bottle cap, see, that Connor found on the floor, and she picked it up and started moving it in her hand. It seemed so easy to do, really not a big deal. It's just that she wouldn't want anyone to see what she'd done, it was none of their business. So if she decided, say, to carve into her leg with the bottle cap and maybe to cut the words "not me" into her thigh, well, she would have to keep covered up, now wouldn't she? I mean, she couldn't then let anybody see her body or let alone be close enough to touch. So she sliced into the leg, her leg, yes it was. And it hurt like bloody hell, but the marks came out good. Course ya can't really tell till the blood goes away, and after slicing in a big red N and then a nice round O…well, the pain overcame the planning. Anyway, "NO" was a pretty good comment, too, yes it was. So she stopped and it burned and she cleaned all the blood. In the light of morning, it was an intense looking wound. But she was pleased. And amazing things occurred.

"Connor cut herself? Or *you* did?" Yes. And yes.

When I went into the bathroom with Cleo, she sat where she sits and we talked like we do, and then when the time came, I could still feel the burning. So I just calmly offered, "I can do this, okay…" and kept rambling on about something else. And I took some toilet paper, was actually surprised at how soft it felt in

118

my hands. And we were fine. Just fine. Cleo didn't mind. And it was done.

At fourteen.

Some people take a while to mature.

"Did she ever say anything about your leg?" No. I don't even think she saw it.

"Not even in the bed? While you slept?" Good question. I honestly don't know. No, she never mentioned it. "Of course she saw it. She must have." I prefer thinking she didn't. I only wrote it for me.

Under really bright lights, the word was legible for well over a decade.

"Your message was to *her*." It really wasn't. I see how you'd think that, but it's kind of a complicated thing. I don't like to write for other people. My words are just for me.

Cleo had this awful sore on her own leg. It was supposedly an ulcer, a vein got poked a long time ago on the edge of a hospital bed. It was actually when her husband was dying and she'd been there late at night, and she stood up too fast, and hit the side of his bed. The damn thing never healed, and she kept it bandaged up and would soak it at night in some hydrogen peroxide solution the doctor told her about. She didn't like doctors, they charge so much and they overreact. There was this open sore just above her ankle for the last thirty years of her life. We all talked about it, of course, and mostly we worried, and she said oh, we shouldn't. She was fine. It was nothing. It was under a bandage of gauze and sometimes it seeped and it looked kinda awful. She didn't want to let Otis see it, when she changed the dressing because he made so much out of things. And Mary Jane, well, that just was not a good idea as one would assume. I asked to see it, well, I was her princess. She said okay and I watched her bathe it, and it wasn't that bad. One would have thought she could find a way to heal it, I guess, but Cleo had things in control, and she just hated

119

hospitals. So she lived with an open ulcer on the side of her leg. For over thirty years. Mostly we pretended it just wasn't there. That worked out well for all concerned.

Dr. Strauss tries to explore if my cutting myself was related to that. Not really, I doubt it. I can see how he'd go there, but hey, can't follow every lead with equal fervor. My family specializes in red herrings.

When the coroner came the night she died, Otis said he asked him about that terrible wound on her leg. So as he mentioned that oh, no, that's just been like that for thirty-two years, the coroner stared at him and looked at the beer and just wrote Otis off as a drunk. It's always so hard to believe what's true if ya haven't been around to watch it transpire.

Everybody's family is odd.
No comment.

"You cut your leg as a protest. It was aimed at her..."
No, I "wrote" in my leg as a reminder to *me*.

- Wash hair.

- Do homework

- Tell Cleo I can clean myself now.

Hey, some people tie a string around the finger. Others draw a little blood.

"Oh, I think you wanted to cut into her..." She didn't *make* me do anything. She was only doing it for *me*, and yes, it was odd, yes, I felt guilty.

"Maybe you felt guilty because of how you felt when she touched you..."

My hair is getting so straggly that Elaine has asked me four times now if I'm trying to let it grow out. No. Just letting it. In a conforming effort to justify my questionable "look" I write and perform a stand-up comedy piece as if I'm a mental patient bag-lady roaming the streets of Manhattan. It's dark, it's clever. Most pleasing is that in many ways, it's true. I say some things out there that I've never told anyone besides Strauss. The high is incomparable.

"So you're really enjoying getting to share some of yourself…" There are days when I think I'll actually be all right.

Any declaration of feeling decent should let me know to soon expect the worst.

Ever gone out to lunch and found you couldn't make it back to your desk? It's a hard one to explain from a payphone.

"What had you been thinking about as you walked down the street?" I know the drill. If I thought this method worked, I'd be happy to play.

The sun was too bright. It's that simple. Things looked edged in an eerie tint, and the glare on mirrored storefronts was nearly blinding. I kept thinking about an old movie with Ava Gardner and dear Mr. Peck called *On The Beach*. The end of the world you see. We've got time for a little sex first, but oh, baby, the radiation is on its way.

"Tell me more…" I'm trying.

"The things she took me to see, my god! I was a little kid and she had me in those movies! No wonder I'm like this!"

"Sure, we know it was bad for you. But that won't help us at this point…what else about *On The Beach*?"

"Now you sound like Mary Jane. Let's just talk about the picture blow by blow and we can pretend I'm Ava Gardner."

"And if we did? Pretend that?"

"We'd all end up dead. They blew up the world, you see." As if my Unconscious is a nudging ghost, I shift in the chair and without warning, my black ripped t-shirt falls off one shoulder. I didn't use to care at all what underwear I had on. Even at Lara's I refused to spend money on elaborate costumes of corsets, garter belts or silk teddies. If they like me, they'll like me in denim, I figured. But today, and oh, okay, *lately*, I've been very deliberate about choosing bras for our sessions. With my new "shipwrecked" look, one never knows when an over-slashed top will stretch off a shoulder, or slide down to deeper cleavage... and if it does, when it does, I don't want to look shabby. Today it's a black silk and lace bra strap beneath my errant shirt. And I put it on for you.

I had to leave the session early. You understand, I hope. I'm so sorry, it's not your fault, it was something to do with Casey, there was a problem and I had to go early today and I forgot to tell you I'm so sorry I'm so sorry.

I go to Blockbuster Videos and rent *On The Beach.*

Those scenes between Ava and Gregory were damned hot for their time.

Connor wonders if Jack ever imagines what her skin feels like. She's seduced lots of men over her years in that hospital, used people right and left. What's one more?

How can I ever tell you that what's been changing lately are my fantasies? Yes, I know Connor is about me, of course I know. But in my mind it's okay to like bad things, humiliating things that I'd never want in life. That's what fantasy is for. Although lately, I've been in bed and without even touching myself I've wondered what it would be like if Connor and Jack actually wanted each other? Not as a game, not as a ploy. But she's an attractive woman and they've gotten close...what if it could happen just once in that scene where the two of them could make love and not just fuck? And which is more humiliating?

I tell people that I have no interest in men anymore now because I had a very wild youth, dated oh, so much and had so much experience as a teenager, that well, I got it out of my system. In a way, it's so true.

We spent most evenings alone, Cleo and I. Well, we shared a bed. There was no other room, it's so simple, really. There was Mary Jane's room and Otis' room and the bedroom that was Cleo's. The choice to let me live had not included an architectural plan. It became mine though, that big room with two doors. Cleo kept her clothes in a front hall closet, saying she didn't want any of her stuff to be in my way. Kids are selfish, for god's sake. It couldn't have occurred to me to say any different. When all was calm on the wacko-front, we'd go to bed early, she and I. Alone in a softly lit sanctuary I tasted how glorious life would've been if we could have lived by ourselves.

"I want to pretend to be Anne from the movie!" And the room was a castle and I was a queen and Cleo could remember dialogue with the best of them. By a 25-watt bulb, we imagined and laughed and hid from everybody. In our bed.

"She met me where I lived, ya see..." *Cleo, please come play!*

"And what did you play?" *Well, when CAN you? I want you now!*

"The poor woman would do anything I said. She and I always acted out parts even when I was real little. I pretended to be Shirley Temple and we'd do scenes from movies we saw on Sunday mornings."

Then I got older, see. And a little older still. *Cleo, I want to do the wedding night again, okay? Where I'm Lenore and you're Walter...*

She cleaned me in the bathroom like I was a little princess, too good to touch such things. I was adored. Don't wish that on me again.

"Why do you think what you did was horrible?" *Excuse me?*

"I used her." I despise the sound of my voice. "It was like Cleo was working at Lara's. They were my fantasies, don't you get it?"

"I hear what you're telling me." He doesn't smile, and I know no joke is nearby. "You were a child. And that's what you keep forgetting. You didn't do anything wrong." Wow. I was way off base – you landed the biggest joke of 'em all.

The true Submissive wants to be absorbed into the Dominant's self – into her body, into her will. He wants a kind of annihilation of his own ego. She matters only, and he is there to be used. There is little feeling of relating. Doing a scene with this kind of "slave" is a lot like being alone with a sex toy.

The true Submissive is also pretty rare.

Instead, what I encountered more often were masochists. Unlike a Submissive, the masochist needs to be the center of attention himself. In fact, he demands it. His pain, his devotion, his humiliation are what matters most. The experience is more than interactive. A long fantasy scene with a masochist can be exhausting. After a while I cringed upon learning that a certain client had made another appointment with me. A little while longer and I grew to almost hate him.

The masochist brings out the sadist in any partner, and his pleasure comes from covertly commanding his own punishment at someone else's hands.

An old joke sums it up pretty well:

"Beat me!" says the masochist.

"No!" says the sadist.

And that's precisely the kind of sadist I was. Resenting, denying, withholding from him everything I knew he wanted. I was not going to be controlled. I refused to get angry and yell at him. I would give him no such satisfaction…in the face of his provocations. I stayed pleasant.

I stayed calm. It was torture.

With most of the clients, I was a delight. They loved me, adored me, and truth be told, they were simply not bad guys at all. Experimenters, players…they came with lots of fantasies and more than enough money, and they asked for a place to be dirty, a place to be naughty. A place to play. Aggressive businessmen, lawyers, CEOs, record producers with strange dark little corners in their minds that screamed for release. Very few of these guys wanted any pain at all; in fact, most were hedonists, complaining if the air conditioning was too low, or the leather too tight. They were eager for bondage and once tied, they liked to be teased and toyed with, used at it were, controlled as it were, until their sexual energy was overtaken by someone else and they were free to simply respond. The games were done in the names of dominance and submission and the roles we played fit those words. But those men were tourists in a very strange land. A lot of the women on staff considered themselves Dominants par excellence and lived that self-image to the hilt, frequenting clubs and bars specializing in their scene. Underneath, most were terrified children of abusive backgrounds who feared their own desires unless they had someone else completely under control.

I said I despised all the men, but I didn't. They were respectful and decent and many were bright and kind of interesting. It's just those masochists who tore the very life out of me, relentless in their need to make everybody else's blood run cold.

No one can touch me. No one will reach me. Any response you see will be a façade. I feel nothing. You're nothing. Fantasy room as microcosm of the world.

Oh, nice - a brand *new* symptom. For the past week, I've been feeling like something horrible is about to happen. A murder, a mutilation. It's like pre-cognition, a psychic's dream. I'm seeing glimpses of some bloody hell to come and I do not when and I do not know who.

"All those attackers are *you*. From inside *you*." Is that supposed to be reassuring?

Casey's gone out of town for five days, and I've agreed to feed and walk her two dogs. Not a problem really. I love those guys, and when we lived together for years I didn't resent taking care of them. Not the way I do with people.

"Now pay attention to that one," Strauss says. "How much you *resent* it when you help. And how it can make you want to hurt yourself. It's not a pure gesture of giving, right? I think you want to show the world the *bloody mess* that love makes." When the man is good, he's good.

It's odd to be in what was once "our apartment" without her around. Like old times. Making myself at home there. No, it was always her house, because deferring to the Taste of Casey was more important to me than any preferences of my own. She'll never find anyone as generous as me, in all definitions of that word. I now wonder if feeling under-appreciated was part of the thrill. It's a huge apartment, should have been room enough for both of us, if, of course, I had actually wanted to be a presence. But all three bedrooms and winding hallway seemed better in her hands. It's not the best of neighborhoods, but for Manhattan, this amount of space is unheard of for our economic range. Most of us mere mortals live in studio shoe boxes, but Casey was always willing to take her chances with the surroundings to have a place large enough for all her stuff. Fears of turning into Cleo, I live light. Not one to keep string. Not one to keep. Dogs are thrilled when I walk in (*Auntie Janine* and all), so I decide to spend the night to keep them company. Mistake.

If I hear one sound in the outside hall, I'm leaping from bed to check the locks. People are crazy these days, violent and angry. For half the night I am convinced I'll be found in a pool of my own blood, surrounded by hungry canines. I try to make it sound amusing. It's actually terrifying. I'm here doing her yet another favor, and I'll be killed for my kindness.

Strauss looks concerned. "So why did you stay there?" Not an altogether bad question.

"The dogs. Hated to leave them up there alone. Animals could be my only weakness. That's why I don't have any." Okay, no comedian gets a laugh all the time.

"You've stopped thinking about getting one yourself?" A dog? No way. God, no. "For a while, I thought ya were." I guess I was just talking. You know how it goes.

As a kid, we had a few "outside" cats over the years. Wild but elegant, when they deigned to come inside, they got highly pampered. Besides good food and warm place to nap, Cleo and Otis offered affection and occasionally we'd hear a validating purr. I wanted to hug them, to explore their beauty, but they were independent and I alone could see it. That calm. And distance. It would be wrong to wreck that calm. The most loving thing was to admire them from across a room. Sometimes I touched my finger to a feline head, just the fur, whispering a touch. But I believed they only tolerated it as the cost of Purina.

"In a way, I did have dogs when Casey and I lived together. I took care of them as much as she did. So, I've already had that experience."

"It's not the same as having your own." I'm sure. But not everyone should be a mom, and no one knows better than me. Then he scrambles in an afterthought, "Now I am not *telling* you to go out and get a dog!" Laughter, and I realize how scary it must be, never knowing what odd command I'm likely to actually obey. "But you said one time that you were *thinking* about it." I know.

"At the time I guess, I figured if I can't ever get myself together, I could at least do something good, like give a dog a really great life."

"Not something you'd do for *you*, huh? Just be doing it for the dog." Why would we think I'm capable of taking care of *anything*?

After a few more rounds, he comes right out with "You're very wrong. You'd make a great mother. Why do you think otherwise?" Okay, all right? Okay, yes, part of me wants to do it. I just don't know. Life is so short, Cleo used to say.

Two months later I carry this tiny puppy into my apartment. *Look around, kiddo. You're home.*

"You've made a choice to have something to love." Well, wouldn't that just thrill you? Let's all pretend I'm only human. Casey is smarter than that and has expressed doubts that I can raise a non-neurotic pet. Fuck you!!! Just...fuck you. I hate the people who think I'm good and kind and I hate the ones who think I'm a mess. Leave me alone.

I name him Pugsley (from *The Adams Family*). Seems appropriate. This commitment is at least proof that I expect to be alive for the next decade. That alone is a rather amazing piece of progress.

I wait till near the end of the session to say it. "Just wondering when maybe you and I should talk about termination." His eyes flash. For god's sake, I was only talking.

"Now?!" he asks. See? I *can* tell when you're really angry. "You want to talk about terminating *now*??" Guess not. Look, hon, it was a friendly gesture. I was offering you a polite way out.

127

I've gotten a little uh, bizarre at work lately. Some of the people think I've gone off the deep end, and it may again, be related to fashion. My entire wardrobe is solid black, and not in that "New York Chic" way. Jeans. T-shirts. Silky skirts. Scarves. All black. No one, not one person in that office has had the nerve to comment. But they sure do watch me. My censors are on vacation, it seems. And I'm having the time of my life. Besides, I want out of there. It would be a relief if they fired me.

"Well you have to do *something* for a living..." I don't want to spend our time discussing career alternatives. I'd like to perform. Or write. Another fantasy.

"I need a break."

"Do you have a large savings?" I have what's in my purse.

Thursday 6 p.m.

"...something happened back there in the bathroom," Strauss says slowly. "Inside your mind. Turning away from your body when you were so over-stimulated, and at the same time, turning on the façade. The two stayed connected. The false smile – and dissociation."

And the *rage*? A word or two on that one, please.

"Probably every bit as stimulating as her touch. And Connor became a way station of sorts, a place to put all those strong feelings. Keeping them, but getting rid of them...at the same time. And at all costs, hiding them from your grandmother."

It's not me.

And in school, hating everyone, hating myself the most.

"And now "school" is your *office*..."

Still hating being seen, being heard. And hating being misunderstood.

"When you first came here, you said the only time you could be yourself was with Cleo..."

The lie. Pretending with her every day of my life. Deceiving both of us.

"*Trying* to, anyway," he adds. "Anything to give her what you thought she needed."

"I was buying her protection."

"Big stakes."

Played out everywhere. Losing myself in Casey, being only what someone else wants.

"And hating them for it…"

Of course.

"Those feelings of *Un*reality," he leans towards me. "I think they were *extreme* reality trying desperately to break through…"

The sun is just too bright. Hyper-clarity.

That day when I was fifteen, walking down the front steps with Cleo. We were heading off to town, a Saturday of nothing but us, me in my thoughts, those funny games…those odd little games where I played like I was someone else…Then a game *within* a game, the nested Chinese dolls, inside my mind a secret kept even from her where Connor and Jack were fighting, were hot for each other…and not from love, not gentleness or praise…those were Cleo's trip, and I secretly had my own…my dominance fantasies for no one's eyes…ever. Cleo pretended to be the man who adored me, and we called each other "darling" while strangers on the bus must have wondered and laughed. I know they watched us, but she swore they did not. I always talked too goddamn loud and no one ever tried to quiet me. Or tone me down. Or let me come. I must have thought the whole fucking world was ME, and no one could overhear or enter this tightly wrapped lie…

Anyway, it was just too bright that day. We shouldn't have gone out at all. So much sun and when it hit my skin, it looked liked strobe lights around my arms. Vibrations and pulsing and lights that could breathe. It can be a kind of seizure, or so Otis said. Flickering followed by highlit shadows, so much like the night that I looked to the moon. Nothing felt alive, not me, not no one. Then everything did, all things inanimate breathed with the light. Not in control of my own brain anymore and it lasted and hours wore on, and we went into town on the bus, but Canal Street had changed. Woolworth's and Holmes had been remodeled, it seemed. New facings, new layers. There were new people working in every store, but that was impossible...nowhere anywhere was anyone the same. Cleo didn't know how to talk to me, it scared her..I never meant to scare her, would die rather than that. Things were so bright that the world itself was melting, and Reality began scraping loose like leaf paint, falling into Canal Street and washing past me...tried to hold my memories, knowing that when the last of it scraped off, there would not be a trace of the world I knew. An oil painting turned into watercolors, and then every figure titled flat as a hieroglyph. We sat in the drug store and ordered sodas while I shrieked inside my mind. The day had simply been too damn bright that morning. No one's fault. Hyper-clarity.

Seeing more than I'd wanted to know.

PART THREE

I look around at our circus of friends, those struggling actors, musicians and such. We're children, all of us, living hand to mouth. We want things so badly, our fame, our success...our prizes. Coming to New York on more than a dream and about a dollar, truly thinking we'll be different. Hey, it does happen. People "make it." They do. It wasn't even me I was rooting for. Every pipe dream was funneled through Casey and I see now that it couldn't have been fair to her. The night I realized she was not likely to ever make it, I cried for hours. Every dream, every hunger would be only that. For years, I was lost in planning a future that was never ours. New York can be an opium den.

There was an 1950's TV game show called *Queen For A Day*. The contestants were highly unfortunate women vying for the title with competing sob stories, each trying to out-pathetic the other in an effort to win prizes and a chance (for one day) to get a make-over and wear a crown. Cleo loved it, and we used to laugh, wondering how the *losers* felt. *Yes, you're tragic, but not tragic enough.* So just go back home still a loser, but without even getting to keep the prize you *came* with. Can't claim to be The Most Pitiful anymore. Talk about robbery.

It's the only intentionally mean thing I've ever said to Casey. She keeps her life in such a bad way, and then expects me to defer because her situation is worse. It always will be and I see that now. I give up, babe. "I'll never win *Queen for a Day* if you're playing!"

My fears of sleeping have progressed to my own apartment. My mattress has been moved to the hall floor, inches from the bolted front door. No one can get in without my instant knowledge. I've had trouble with these feelings, but never this bad. I can't believe what's happening to me anymore. What an irony if after it all, I'm even crazier than I thought.

Monday 6 p.m. *(But it could be Thursday, it could be Friday – time itself is no longer mine).*

"Let's look at this head on today" he puts down the pad. Just us. All that attention. No one deserves it. "I may have a few ideas about where that fear comes from…"

"I've never been harmed, never. This is not some trauma that I've repressed. Why would I be so terrified of being attacked?"

"Maybe you're not. Maybe it represents something else." Watching me, talking carefully. He doesn't know if I'm ready to go there. Only since last session have I started to think about it. When my shirt fell off my shoulder, I started to see. I think of us, of you, of Jack of Connor of who the hell is who anymore….that's part of it, isn't it? No one will ever break through. Or get in. Or come inside me. Literally. The desire I feel when I sit in this room with you is more than I can take. You are just an ordinary man. You're nothing. It is not me.

Yes, I dress to arouse you. Yes, sometimes I imagine seducing you. And other times, I imagine you reaching first. So shoot me.

"You know me," I say quietly. "All about me. Yes, I've thought it, that if I'm ever going to experience sex, real sex, it should be with you. At least, you could take me as me."

"All very logical, huh?"

"Okay, okay. Yes. Occasionally I've had sexual thoughts about you. About us. Everybody does, right? In therapy, its part of the transference…"

"We're talking about…"

"Me. Yes. I got it… So I have, okay? Yes, I've wondered what it could feel like if you touched me, my body. And different fantasies.."

"What kinds of fantasies?" I cannot do this.

"Look, I've told you how we all try to charm. My mother and Cleo, it's how we operated. They seduced, not literally, well sometimes. It kept us safe. Men are dangerous, ya need the upper hand, to be in control and it's like Lara's and what I did there, I mean what I was trying to do here I guess. I'm sorry."

"No need to be sorry. You can think and say anything here, without any action resulting. Right? But still believe if you act

132

seductive, I'll be seduced. If you're angry, you'll destroy us. Not true."

"Sorry.." I hear it. "Noooo... nevermind. *Everything's fine.* Is that better?"

"Uh, that's "Sorry's" sneaky cousin." And still playful. I was afraid that saying any of this would change you. Us. Sterilize us. "Just *maybe* this relationship is sturdier than you've thought!" What if nothing is?

In the darkly-lit back attic of my brain, I allow myself to wonder. Did you buy it? The tale that I want to seduce you only for power? That it's all been strategy within my control? After all this time, will you swallow a lie?

Pugsley The Dog sleeps on a pillow right next to my head. The sound of his breathing is incredible, but there is another sound that means even more. He sighs just as he's stretching out and relaxing right before sleep. A long heavy sigh. Trust. I understand that sound from the inside out.

The way you look at me sometimes, Sir Strauss. Into me. Almost with affection. Do you forget for awhile that I'm this filthy mad-child? All the things I've done and told, they should make you squirm with revulsion. For god's sake even my own goddamn father never wanted his eyes to rest on my face! But sometimes...yours almost seem happy there.

It's one thing to be caught in a loveless marriage, but poor Cleo didn't even love her lover. Mr. Clay was nice, Mr. Clay was attentive. She talked about him as if he was an applicant whose positive qualitics she was judging for job suitability. There was shame of course, after the fact. She should never have done it. She was foolish and she didn't even want to, she just did, not sure why. I never cared and wouldn't have condemned her, but she was nearly destroyed by a passionless affair, and even to jaded me, that seemed sad. Women really don't have sexual feelings though, she explained. We're just made to love our children.

I watch Casey and her parade of boyfriends. No woman is really happy, and men can only be satisfied temporarily. The guys at Lara's were the easiest to please. At least they were sure what they wanted.

The thought has occurred to me that it'd be a shame to die without ever knowing what it feels like. An experiment of sorts. But I've never thought I could do it without leaving the room. I was hardly present with my clients. They were there and I heard them, but feelings flew like birds in migration. We're late, hurry, catch up to the flock. Move it!!!

But this man, this doctor – I honestly believe I could touch him and stay present. I know I could. It's already happened.

The second year of my treatment we got into an argument about his vacation. Not the fact that he was leaving me; I couldn't care less. Well, *then* I couldn't. But at the end of the last session before he was going away, he put out his hand and said "have a good summer." A perfunctory little handshake that was basically a patronizing effort at caring. I know. He's said it before. I'm harsh. But I told him all that when he finally returned. Over time more vacations came up, and we merely said "see ya" with no hand offered at all. Wouldn't it seem I'd be pleased?

"Because you don't even shake hands with me anymore when you go away…"

"What?!" That reaction does not encourage free association, doctor "You told me you thought it was impersonal. Don't you remember?"

"Yeah, I said it seemed that way. I didn't say we shouldn't do it anymore though." It's moments like these that make me positive he either despises me or is a true masochist. "I guess now that you know so much about me… last time, when you didn't even offer, it was easy to think its because I'm so repugnant in your eyes…" I can't remember how many sessions we danced with this one. I only remember where it led.

"I'm wondering," he offers carefully "if your cutting yourself is related to sexual feelings at all. You have affectionate thoughts in here, and then you call me and say you want to hurt yourself…" I want to know that you don't despise me, that's all. Only that. Is that just too much to need?

A lot of the submissive men at Lara's were searching for a safe place for their desire. Under the sharp heels of a woman with a whip probably doesn't seem like the best spot to look, but the game of dominance and submission is about exactly that - containment of dangerous passions, and any strong partner offers the greatest of solace. Control me, he begs. Confine me. Put borders around my longing and grant me only as much pleasure as you choose. Now my urges can't run away with us, because you won't let them. Make me do it all for you, and I'm finally safe enough to feel.

Thursday 5:40.

"So I guess I can't be satisfied," I'm in such a deadened mood. Trying to make logical leaps. Even my arguing lacks punch today. "That's what I'm supposed to say, right? I mean, clearly, I know what the right answer is..."

"No, ya don't," Strauss answers fast. Does he match my moods as I used to think? Or maybe he's just him. "See, we're not after any right answers here, so there *isn't* one." Sorry, but Cleo had an answer to that, too. *That's what people will tell you to trick you saying what you think.* – from The Stone Tablets of Grandma

By the time Mary Jane had been to the hospital for the third time, Cleo had the experience down to a science. Well, her science. And there were things she could do to help. Psych ward emergency rooms churn out some provocative questions when interviewing any new guest.

What's your name?

Do you know what day it is?

What year?

These, of course, procure insights into the lucidity of would-be patient. But there might also be a more in-depth query.

Who's the president of the United States?

Okay, reasonable enough.

And the Vice-President?

Under extreme anxiety, it's easy to draw a blank on this one.

Can you name the Secretary of State?

Yep, that's the show-stopper. And it terrified poor Cleo.

Truth is, they're not expecting correct answers. The question is designed to show how a patient responds to *not* knowing. Does the anxiety make her angry? Manic? Does she become delusional in the face of confusion and offer answers like "I am the President" or "Frank Sinatra is"? If a response like that comes up, the questions may continue with "and who's your senator?" to follow the thread of the patient's imagination. But when Cleo heard all of it, she formed an unmovable theory of her own. Mary Jane had been labeled "schizophrenic" merely because she filled in the blanks with movie stars. They (the Establishment) valued politics higher than Hollywood, and so they used current affairs as indicators of normalcy. Hence, if her dear nervous daughter was to be seen as healthy enough to get out of the hospital quick, she would need to walk in there armed with all the Right Answers.

--- Diagnostic & Statistical Secrets Uncovered Only By Cleo

From then on, when she went to the store to pick up movie books and National Enquirer and Racing forms she started adding Newsweek and Time to the shopping cart. During dinner we studied, practiced and actually used homemade flash cards. Whenever Mary Jane started acting a little more peculiar than usual, Cleo shifted into high gear and fired away like were studying for finals.

"The secretary of defense?...Okay, how many members in Congress?... what's the president's wife's name..."

It could be argued that all those pop quizzes actually encouraged the next hospital visit, because Mary Jane was desperate to be seen as an obedient student and always cooperated to her fullest. For many years, even in the depths of her darkest psychosis, she could still rattle off the names of every cabinet member.

Things got more complex when a new resident on staff decided to add a splash of old sayings.

"Can you tell me what the following mean?

A bird in the hand is worth two in the bush.

People in glass houses shouldn't throw stones..."

Our Little Red Schoolhouse of rote memorizing suddenly became a graduate seminar.

"...because stones can shatter glass." Otis was always one for the obvious.

"No, honey," Cleo was edgy. "I mean, yes, they can, but there has to be more to it. See, they *mean* something. Mary Jane?"

"Not to cause trouble, I guess," Mary Jane's eyes darted around the room as she talked. "If you don't want more trouble, then don't throw them." Not right, but not totally awful. Cleo graciously accepted any remotely creative response. "But that bird one is hard. It's easy to hold one bird, easier than two, but you don't think so..."

"It's so *simple*, Mary Jane," Otis got better at the game with a few beers in him. "It's about security. You don't want to lose your security!"

"That's good, honey!" smiled grandma. The world was right. "Mary Jane, can you see what he means?"

A rolling stone gathers no moss nearly did us all in.

"Mama, moss is a fungus!" Otis yelled and winced. "That IS crazy. Nobody in their right mind wants a fungus." Even though I was supposed to stay out of it unless everyone else got stumped, my patience had thinned.

"It means anyone on the go!" I hollered. "Always on the move for God's sake! It's got nothing to do with moss!!!"

"But it's a *good* thing to put down your roots."

"Not if you're near a fungus..."

"It's not good or bad, it's just an observation..."

"You can't roll forever..."

To this day, I haven't a clue what the damn thing means.

Dear Miss Bartchey,

Please excuse Janine from school for the rest of the week. There's just too much to talk about here...

I watched a highly mediocre film on TV last night, and this man and woman were dancing…a huge ballroom, haunting waltz, and the two of them. It could have been *any* movie, hardly memorable. But at the end of that scene I knew I'd never forget it. Two characters, while their bodies moved together, had looked *into* each other's eyes, and yes, of course, what a tired old phrase, but they *were* **honestly** looking *into* each other… faces tilted, eyes locked like flirting children, nearly giggling from the trance of their mutual stare. Looking into someone else's self. Showing while seeing. Hinting, then promising that "I really do know what you feel, and *more*. I also know that *you* know that I know…" and smiles warm as fire.

I used to think *gazing* was about something else.

I was good at flirting, or I think I was. But I didn't really get it.

Nothing's new under anyone's Sun, but last night was the first time I understood what people feel.

I'm actually reading *Ulysses*. Well, Joyce more than anyone can take my mind off myself. Years ago, I picked up a copy of *Dubliners* and *Portrait*… and although I was captivated, I also knew that someone not perfectly educated couldn't appreciate what was on such a page. There are other books to read in conjunction, and then essays and literary criticism…one day, I figured, maybe I'd have time, or energy. Maybe when/if I wasn't so scared of truly immersing myself….I guess one day after I turned into somebody *else*, I'd be ready. Then dressed in a bride's lingerie, I'd hold a thick bound version of a genius mind and let him in.

Don't think about yourself so much. I used to swear I couldn't help it, that oh, poor me, couldn't turn it off. Lately at least I'm realizing I probably could. I just don't want to.

When Joyce writes a day of Mr. Bloom, it's not events that matter. The inner world, the repeated thoughts, connected by the thread of mind alone. The way we think plunked down in a novel. Beyond a PET scan, beyond any psych unit. Inside the human mind.

My intellectual bent is the one thing they couldn't touch. Yes I could play sexual games, yeah I let her wipe me in the bathroom, I argued and laughed and whined and screamed along with the rest of the barnyard. But they did not read Joyce. Sometimes I wonder if my father was a genius.

"You're having thoughts about your father lately?" Oh, I can see the glee. Strauss thinks its remarkable that I never wondered about ol' dad, didn't ask questions, never fantasized. With everything about me, oh, yeah, let's call me "odd" because of that one. The man simply didn't matter. The last thing I wanted was another relative.

"He crosses my mind, yeah. Probably because you try to bring him up every so often."

"Doing it for me."

"You flatter yourself."

"It wasn't *me* who brought *me* up."

I did a drawing of you the other night, charcoal, several shades. It's you, this room, and me – or the me from long ago. I'm in the middle of the floor with a small fence around me in a circle, kind of like the Unicorn Tapestries, enclosed in a pen, but mine is made of barbed wire. There are cuts on my arms and legs, I've pulled the fencing close to me, protecting me. Or you? You stand there with an outstretched hand, gentle smile, seemingly unimpressed with the droplets of blood on your floor. We just stand, you and me. My face is far away, your eyes are open and warm. Part of my body is hidden behind furniture, part of my foot has slid under the rug. Part of.

There are nights where I imagine you holding me.

There are days in that room when I simply wish we could touch.

"I'm only asking for a handshake." I implore, close to tears. "For connection. When I get so scared, sometimes the thought of you making contact with me, helping me feel grounded…if you'd touch my hand."

"You're forgetting the reality here, forgetting *me* – that I am a separate person. Touching would be a violation of this relationship. It's not part of the way I work here, and you *know* that somewhere in there…"

"Even if it'd make me feel like you don't despise me? Like you could stand me…"

"When I go away next month, if you want me to shake your hand, I will. But your insistence that I physicalize our relationship, we need to keep talking about all this."

"It's such a simple thing really. I mean, I actually thought you'd be pleased that I want any kind of comfort."

"No, it's far from simple. Your *conflict* about touch means its not – wouldn't be a pure gesture. It could be very damaging to your treatment."

Silence. And the hour's almost gone.

"What are ya thinking?"

"Hating myself. The same fucking thought as always…" Soft words, eyes down. I'm such a goddamn sick thing.

"Hating yourself because you feel rejected? Can you see what's happening here today?" Silence as art form. "Stay with me," he says. "You created this situation. I'm right here with you, listening attentively. But *touching* has no part in this treatment. And you know that. In a few days I'm going away, and I made a big mistake by not telling you at the right time last session. All things that you have no control over. So you *create* a situation by wanting physical contact from me, and predictably, I say no - but maybe that's not clearly rejecting *enough* - to justify how angry you feel, so you ask again and again till I get adamant and lay it all out firmly. Well, then you're off and running, getting to hate yourself because you think you've ruined our relationship. You *walked in* here today hating yourself and feeling helpless, so you created this scene where you *were* in control – you *caused* this rejection. As if you were pushing me away, making me leave…and that took away your feelings of having no control in the situation."

Mostly, I hate that I want you. I lived a good long life without ever feeling anything like this. I despise us both.

"You hate wanting, longing. It makes you furious..."

Later Pugsley and I take a very long walk. Strolling along the river, then past your office just to see if the light in the window is still on. But I start to feel guilty, like I'm just *using* His Dogness for my sneaky little plan. We stop at Petland on the way back. It's a multi-treat night.

When we sleep now, he's still on the pillow next to me, but lately he's moved closer, and he presses his warm body against the side my head. Keeping contact through the night. I try to stay completely still so he won't move away. Sometimes he looks at me and I could swear he's saying "Jeez. Chill. You're trying too hard."

Strauss adds "When Pugsley lies right next to ya, it's *partly* for himself..." No really, that's the remarkable part. I didn't put him there, it's something he does on his own. "Right," Strauss smiles. "And... it's partly for *himself.*"

With a dog, you can be who you are. Clearly, I knew that going in. The surprise is not that I don't have to pretend around Sir P. What's amazing is that I'm usually in a *good* mood with him. Euphemism. I'm downright silly in his presence.

We are all so goddamn *loud*, my family. Intense. We were all so embarrassingly intense.

"The part of you that's playful, teasing, sexual. You say that's all in fantasy, that's all Connor. Connor is part of *you*. What is it about her that you're so afraid to let me see?"

Casey was going to be a superstar and I would've been the reason. A monstrous home in the hills, that's what Star-Makers deserve. Hundreds of wanna-bees would try to contact me, hoping to meet, wanting to hear me proclaim that they had "It" and could succeed. See, I was not meant to have this meaningless life. We were gonna be stars.

Well, it was by far my sanest fantasy. At eighteen, I thought I could discover the secret to alchemy, and it would be more than turning iron into gold. Language, bodies, life itself could be transformed. The Secrets of the Ages would be written in my brown leather book. I would be a professor of science and no one could understand me until I found those secrets and the world would be mine.

I was a child queen and literally ran the house. Growing up was bound to be an anti-climax.

There were books I would write, or so I hoped when I was seventeen. Not many kids in public high school could even make it through *Portrait of The Artist...*, let alone write a decent essay on the work.

What a wunderkind I was.

What a waste.

I don't even know anyone who realizes that James Joyce changed the way the modern novel was written. And not only that, he altered the way we think. Stream of consciousness and fragments of interconnecting images came into our shared mental processes when *one man* wrote a book. My god. My god. Linear order marshaled our philosophies and our psyches for centuries, and no one I know even wonders how that changed.

This rage is unbearable, and in the next second, I say no it's not, it's perfect. I have never felt more me. Just STOP IT! All of you, everyone stop trying to change me, to fix me up like something you bought at a fucking yard sale, and you think I might work well for ya, so you put in some effort. I was not yours to buy and I'm not yours to use! Leave me the fuck alone and go work on yourself!!

Casey cares about me. Yes. Yes. Yes. She tries to fix me up to suit herself. A pick here, a remold there. LEAVE ME ALONE. I DO NOT BELONG TO YOU.

What do we human beings do to each other in the name of help?

This will benefit you. You'll be better if you try this. Here, just for you. Because I care. I know what works.

I DO NOT BELONG TO YOU!

Thursday 5:30.

"What are ya thinking?" he asks as he often does if I just sit there, silent, cryptic. Seductive. As if I'm never more appealing that when a million miles away.

"Jack and Connor fantasies again..." Abstract enough for ya?

"What kinds of thoughts?"

"Us. I mean, yes, fantasy characters. But sometimes it is you and me...we don't need to go into it for god's sake."

"Nope. Don't need to. But it could be useful."

"I know how uncomfortable this makes you. I'm sorry."

"Not uncomfortable. Not *me*, anyway," and shakes his head. "You do this a lot, right? We've talked about it. Trying to get me to *make* you tell me something."

"Maybe that's part of the fantasy..." If I do look right at you, and you swear you're not uncomfortable, how do I keep trusting a liar? "It's not awful or anything. Just personal... I don't know..."

"Stay out here. Don't go off inside your mind..."

"That is what I want, yes. Okay, it's become erotic to me, is that what you want to hear?"

"And what's that anger about?"

"Guess."

"Or you could tell me."

"I imagine us fighting, arguing. You want to hear? I'm not the one who's uncomfortable about it." Silence. Not forcing. Not playing. Yeah, I get it. "That I'd start to head for the door, fight with you, you'd grab me and hold me...we'd both want each other. Yes, a sexual fantasy, okay? And on that couch, that I never sit on, that couch we've never touched...you'd hold me and I'd try to fight you...and you'd understand that I wanted you to kiss me. But I won't tell you I do. And you're playful, but serious...and you refuse. You say something like "oh, no, I'm not gonna make you a victim here. If you want me, say so, little girl. You can't have this without saying you care..." and I hit at you

143

and you smack me playfully...but you won't kiss me unless I say it...tell you I want you, that you reached me, that you matter..."

He listens only. And tries to keep watching. They're only words, I know that. But they're mine.

He's cautious when I get ready to leave today. Still watching, wondering if I'm likely to go off and hurt myself now. He asks "you okay there?" and smiles such an unprotected smile as if he's saying "hey, you in there...it's not awful. And ya know it. Stay in reality on this, and let's talk some more..."

The world does look different some days. There's a pink tree, cherry blossoms I guess, and after Monday's evening session I usually walk along the river... and whenever I see this tree with its pitch black trunk, I realize it's more vivid than anything I ever thought up in my head. I've imagined that Connor's window is above the tree, that she watched it change through season after season, while she stays the same, in the hospital, waiting. For death probably. Getting out had simply never occurred to her. She's always known she was crazy.

At this point, there are just so many nice little choices. I'd slice my wrists, or I'd eat or I'd vomit or I'd starve or I'd hit or I'd cry or I'd die. Or I'd panic or I'd drink or I'd shriek or I'd hate or I'd split or I'd shit or I'd suck or dismember, depersonalize, delude, deny - or hear a voice or see a sight and sleep too much or never snooze or go out on a ledge or hang by an edge, and no one believes in green eggs and ham. Oh, doctors, dearies, don't spend too much energy caring about the symptom. *Any* would do. Just pick something from the Tree of No-Ledge and start up an illness. It's probably about the same things underneath. The "disorder" may be nothing but a mirage, all smoke and mirrors, giving us a place to hide while we say what we lack the guts to say without the code of illness. If the name doesn't matter, the DSM assignation is the biggest red herring going. It's about longing and needing and the fear that our feelings are so strong they'll literally kill us. Period. That, my chickies, is the heart of Mental Illness, all Axii included. The rest is window dressing.

I don't WANT a normal life! I want what's inside me cut out, sliced clean. Get it out like a demon, or an unwanted child.

Kill it and take it and even fucking Rosemary didn't have to raise her own wicked baby!!!!

Of all the things I ever thought, the best is this – I am not equipped to be in charge of a life. A horrendous mistake has been made.

IF YOU CAN'T FIX ME, STOP TRYING TO TAME ME.

It's all just speeches and cream. The lingo, the dance. We'll talk and see what helps. No one has ever understood.

Telling some things are embarrassing. Others, downright mortifying.

Pugsley and I have a game we made up together. He rolls onto his back and suddenly there is this perfectly rounded, pudgy belly covered in soft gold hair. It's one thing to rub and scratch it. But I decided he needed a little background music. Now when he hears me sing it, he shows his belly and wiggles till its touched.

Puppy-tummy time is early
Puppy-tummy time is late
Puppy-tummy time is the middle of the day
Puppy-tummy time starts at eight
Any ol' time is Puppy-tummy time
When you see a tummy this great!

Well, *Pugs* doesn't think its stupid.

Too much is happening and it's happening too damn fast. Words and looks in that room with you, ideas and memories. I understand so much of it. I see it. But it doesn't help enough.

"So we keep working. And hopefully you'll find something that *will*."

It's all in the hands of the mental patient. What an interesting concept.

"There's a cartoon I'm thinking of," Strauss smiles. "...from The New Yorker, maybe, I don't remember. A prisoner is standing on a road, dressed in his prison stripes, with a heavy ball and chain tied around his ankle. But the chain has been cut in half; he's free - the ball lies on the ground but its no longer attached to his leg. He looks down at it with this perplexed look on his face and says: "So, what am I supposed to do NOW?!"

We all like to know who we are.

I'm the girl who has to pretend.

A few details about Lara's. Things unsaid till now. "It's time I told you something, to really help you see..."

"Ya mean like a veil behind a veil behind a veil?" If I take my eyes off the floor, I know you'll be grinning. I am, ya know, getting to actually know you. "A mask behind a mask?" Okay, okay. Have I cried "Der Wolfe!" a bit too often?

"*All* of it is you," he says. "You're one person, a very complicated person, but ... you're... *you*." Then he laughs. "There – the psychiatrist finally sums it up for ya. You're you. How's that for technique?"

And you're you. Within the past year, that's gotten clearer. You've let me know who *you* are, too, and it makes no sense why that should be helping, but it is.

"I'm gonna blind him, Mama!" Otis is standing in the hallway, talking towards the corner. "That no good son-of-a-bitch had no right to look at me that way! I could get him in the eyes, it's the worst you know, to live blind! The goddamn bastard couldn't walk down the street after I finish with him!!!" His rage makes his body shake, and she stands near him, listening, waiting it out as if he's having some kind of seizure. She knows it's not, but she also knows it has to come out. And for all the times she shushes and silences I hear her now in the darkness of a corner, alone with him as she's alone with each of us, letting him rave...no, more than that – she's throwing him bones.

"Oh, you could hurt him, honey, if you wanted to. I know you could finish him off." And her son shakes more and he pounds one fist into the other. He knows he has to hurry and get it over with. She won't let him talk that way when we come any closer. "You could kill him, or you could maim him. Either one..." And no one but him has ever heard her talk like this. Secret languages, we all have them, but she's so multi-lingual and I never never knew.

"Oh, Janine, honey..." she says in our bed. "You know how silly those two can be. You understand everything, my princess... Anne? Did you want to play like Anne, or somebody else?"

And those government plots. How many of those did she uncover with her daughter? They talked alone, too, and it must've been in code. "I understand what you saw, Mary Jane" she whispers once. "I know. You know I do..." Feeding each of us a little of what we crave. Playing roles in our scripts, playing along. That word. Let's play. Play with me. We're only playing.

And it's been the wrong word.

Playing takes two. Two people discovering. Two people creating together. Not one person pulling all the strings.

She was working me.

Monday/Thursday
5:00
6:00
Timeless.

"I think that's been hard for you here," he says, "...our playing. You like it, but it's been *new*. The back and forth. Not knowing what I'd say..." Ooo, baby. That is definitely the key phrase. Before you, I preferred my conversations scripted. Memorized. No improvising allowed.

"Cleo, he won't drink anymore, right? He said he'd stopped drinking after last time…"

"That's right, honey. He said he could see that it wasn't good. He won't drink anymore. That's over." Tell me again, please. "He stopped for good." Thank you.

We know its not true. We know. We're not stupid. What's the old joke?

A man gets a flat tire on the street next to a mental hospital. As he changes the tire, the four lug nuts fall free and roll down a drain where he can't retrieve them. He makes a fist and curses and thinks and thinks but can't find a way to drive his car without the four bolts to fasten on the tire. A mental patient stands watching on the other side a high fence and suddenly says "calm down fella, why don't ya just take one bolt from each of the other three wheels and then all of 'em would have three. That's enough to hold your tires on."

"Wow, thank you!" says the amazed man on the outside. "Incredible! I would never have thought of that! How could YOU come up with it?!!"

Excuse me," says the indignant lunatic. "I'm in here because I'm crazy, not stupid."

Tell me the story again, Cleo. Tell me I'm who I want to be. And when I ask if it's all true, lie again, Cleo. Please lie again. Thank you. There is no one, no one like you in all the world through eternity.

But you were never supposed to be working ME. I was yours, I was Janine. Your cohort. Your lady. Your princess. You would never have worked me, would you?

"She monitored all your bodily functions?" Yeah, well she took care of me, saying I shouldn't have to do all that, and she swore she didn't mind. She loved me too much. She got pleasure in helping…

"I'm sure she did love you - very much." His voice is soft. "But it was *not* all for you. And I think you see that now." She

148

loved loving me, yes. She got pleasure in taking care of me. "It's more than that." I know.

"I despise my body. The fact that I exist in the visible world. All I ever wanted was to be a ghost, an *idea*. I want to be Pure Thought, not flesh, not something people can mock and measure. I am not here for other people! And I'm tired of you telling me to give people a chance. All the pretending, all the bullshit I've put on for everybody else and not one fucking person appreciates it! I want them to see it! To hear and feel and breathe along with me and finally know what I go through for them! How I try to hide everything they don't like, try to live and look normal for them. To see how much I love them, how much I've given!!!"

"To see what, now?" LISTEN to me!

"How desperately, literally desperately, I love them!"

"Look at your hands..." My fists. I unclench and am shaking again. "Yes, I'm furious, so what?! Because I want them to realize what a goddamn hero I've been!"

"One more time. How much you love them?"

"What do you want me to say? That I hate them? Yes! By now I do fucking hate them!"

"Always have." Always have. "And hate pretending."

"Yes! That's what I've been saying for as long as I've been here! I hate having to pretend!"

"Who's been making you?" All of them! "*Nobody* is making you pretend except you."

"But why would I do that to me?"

"To stay safe. You get to say oh, look what everyone makes me do. Then you pull away. No danger of getting too close, not if ya believe everyone is a vulture!"

Perennial victims provoke their abuse. They stay hurt, mistreated and it comes with a perk – a free ticket to hate, no guilt attached. Well, who wouldn't despise an abuser? Victims are not sadistic, poor lambs. They only hate because of what someone else did to them.

149

To say they're all making me do it. Shoving masks on my face. Tying my hands with pretty ribbons of lies. I pretend with everyone and then despise them for it.

Or

I start out hating. And then I pretend.

"I think you start out fearing them, then the anger, then pretense."

"Fearing what? In some ordinary boring little person?"

He laughs. "Well, no there's not much to fear if you think no more of them than that!"

"I'm afraid around you sometimes."

"I'm not a very scary guy." Yes. You are. And I sort of see.

"Never once, never..." he insists, "have I ever said you have to be a certain way here. You've pretended I did...."

"I can't help it then, I have no choice but to always wear a mask..."

"You've thought ya needed them, but it sure wasn't aimed at *pleasing* people. *Having* to wear masks was a way to prove to yourself that everyone is just too damn demanding.. So who needs 'em? Who'd want 'em? Not you. You've seen what they make you do, so you don't put up with anyone for very long. Look at what *they* do to you...you wouldn't love anyone like that. So you can't have needs. Won't have longing. Won't want anybody. Who'd want THEM?"

Who'd want YOU? (Oh, teacher, can you see my raised hand?)

One day a month or so ago, I bumped into you on the sidewalk right before a session. You were getting out of a cab, and probably coming from home, right out of the shower. Anyway, your hair was still wet at the ends, and as you walked ahead of me through the door I saw the damp hair against your skin on back of your neck. I was careful to walk close, watching

150

you. You looked so real at that second, so human. There was a time when I might have smirked at you for running late, barely having time to shower... I might have thought *oh, the great wizard is just mortal.* And if I'd had such a thought, I'm sure you would've heard about it. That is not the thought I had. I wanted to kiss you, to feel the moist hair, to taste your skin. I wanted you to hold me against your chest and touch my hair with your lips. I wanted you to nuzzle me the way Pugsley does, to rub your face across my own, to play. With neither of us pulling any strings, I wanted your body to play with mine.

Otis owned a gun, and although Cleo swore he never had bullets, there were so many lies that surely, gunpowder would have been included. He didn't get angry that often, he didn't go out that often, and only "out there" could someone say something mean. Only out there were people truly dangerous and heartless and the kind (you know the kind) who would pick on somebody or try to take advantage. The kind who had to be stopped.

Mr. Jergens was only the owner of a little grocery, not some powerful enemy, and certainly no demon. He could be rude, oh, sure, he was curt and although it's not the end of the world, he might not have liked us very much. Otis had a run-in with him, on one day one fall day. That Mr. Jergens was a mean man, and we all said that maybe he was. But to think he had to be gutted, that he had to be sliced open from the belly down and have his intestines ripped out...to hear how he would die, with internal organs bleeding upon themselves, the agony was guaranteed if he was left someplace where no one could find him, and the bleeding is slow but more than slow is the pain of every nerve from the intestinal track exposed to air and sliced down the middle. The damage would be done with knives and a hammer, the gun was only to get his attention while they drove someplace quiet. Autumn is such a pretty time of year, and when I look at leaves that's what I think of.

Nothing bad ever happened. Every day Cleo reminded me that he never hurt anybody, and it was only talk. But he was so so loud and so so angry. And the tremble of the house itself when he ran down the hall, the vibration of the windows when he flung open that cedar closet where she let him keep his gun...it was just so loud. I know sounds can't kill. Not in a bloody way. I know. And after a while, when its all in your mind (and really what isn't?), after a while it all just fucking may as well have happened. For all the same its remembered.

"As terrifying as that must have been, there is a very big difference between a man who talks like that and someone evil." NO. You would like to think it, because it keeps your world nice. I never liked flowers in a row. They're meant to grow wild and if you're gonna tame them and put 'em behind your fence, at least let them grow as they fucking grow! Leave them *something*.

Monday 6:40 p.m.
"My life, my family..." I feel we're at some cut-off point, me and Strauss. "They were not the worst, you know. I mean some people have *terrible* parents, but they don't grow up to be as crazy as me..."

"Sounds like you're wondering what part you play in it all."

"I guess. And mostly why the craziness went on for so damn long..."

"Nothing in your house was ever outgrown, right?" Pretty good there, doctor. "Keeping everything forever." Every card, every toy, every box. "I think you've also been keeping your family in much the same way. In your fears. Every word of theirs interlaced through your own thoughts – a way of keeping them literally alive."

"We all do that, though. I mean, we all carry a past around..."

"Most of us carry it in *addition* to ourselves. Not *instead* of..." We sit in the quiet and the sunlight outside gets weaker. His office faces the river and orange lights flutter across the rug at this time of day. How apropos for a therapist to occupy a room that actively shows a passing of time.

"I've been getting afraid it will start up again – the cutting." My head is down, asking *please be easy with me*.

"*It* will?" I don't care for the tone. "You make it sound like weather. It's raining today. It's hot, it's cold..." Oh, this may not be the treatment of my dreams, you know. It just might be, however, the best of the real world.

"Okay, okay," I half-smile. "Did I mention that I'm thinking about cutting myself again?"

"*Much* better." And I go on to tell you how those self-inflicted wounds don't even help anymore. The last time I did it with any fervor was a day you cancelled cause you were sick. I'd taken the day off from work, not out of worry, not out of terror, but for me. Because I wanted the day. I jogged in the park that morning, cold left-over snow, I had to run carefully, but anything was worth the sight of those frosted trees, the dark London-type skies, the crisp air...it was cold, but not frozen. Cool but not ice. And I thought about getting to talk with you, thought about having the morning to stay myself, to not have to be around those "others" and not having to mask it up, and I thought about you and wondered if you jog and I stopped off for a take-out breakfast, well, I had to bring home some bacon to share with my life-mate. And when I walked back in the door, the message light was on and you were sick with a cold and you wouldn't meet with me today. And all of it, the ice and the cold and the beauty and the plans and all of my stupidity and all of the longings ("yeah, *there's* the word!") just made me reach for the plastic take-out fork and stab into my arm. Pugs looked confused and I stopped right away, wouldn't ever stop for a human, but hey, dogs are peculiar things. I looked at my arm and I felt not as good as I should, and it seemed like yesterday's news and I understood a bit more. Besides you'd just say I was doing it to show you, to aim the fork at you. It might be on its way out, this cutting. I found a bandage, and rinsed the gash and again, felt not ecstatic, or terrified or debased, but kind of annoyed. No, not with a bang, but it might be whimpering its way out of usefulness.

I always hated it when people bought little cute coats for their pets. Like they give a fuck what somebody thinks and need to parade like everybody parades...oh, who cares? I got him a gray fleece coat because it's cold outside. It's not plaid or flowered or anything stupid. But it's cold out there and he loves to go walking.

153

One of the coolest Freud quotes is "There comes a moment when the analyst loves the patient, and the patient knows it and is cured." Cool in sentiment, anyway. What kind of cure occurs if a patient fears she's hated?

"Why would ya need to think such a thing?" He shows little emotion with it. That's part of the problem, maybe. He won't tell me anything about how he feels. If he can stand me. And if anyone could.

"It helps me to feel safer, I guess. Because you won't tell me... If I could know that you still have any compassion for me...at all." (It's pure bullshit. I'm fishing and I'm ready to go deep sea diving. Who the fuck *wouldn't* hate me?)

The session is spent. Maybe we both are. Then in his inevitable 11th hour save, Strauss gestures to the clock. "We need to stop in a minute. But listen... you know I care about you – very much. And I think you *know* that." It's strange, how tense he looks. Uncomfortable in his own chair. Well, I've left him little room to move.

I'm instantly sorry for all this. He's clearly no happy camper, but keeps talking. "There is nothing about you that repels me, not at all. And you know *that* as well." I nod. Only. "I feel the need to say this today because of how harsh you've been with yourself lately, of how you can treat yourself. But I'm certainly not wild about having to. And it *doesn't serve* you...."

I do know you care. But it's hard to keep knowing once I walk home.

"You're not gonna like this," he starts in early on me. "because you never do..." I appreciate his warning though. "If you want to feel loved by someone - you could have that kind of relationship. You could find someone to love you." Stop it. I am so sorry I ever brought up the entire idea. I've done my share of providing the world with orgasms. "We're talking about *love*."

STOP IT.

Mary Jane liked oral sex, she thought it could feel good if a man kissed her down there. Oh, thank you so much for sharing.

See, it wasn't that Cleo and I did sexual acts for god's sake. We played little fantasy games and pretended to be different people, yes I know I've said that before. We acted things out. That's all. And sometimes when we laughed at how silly people were when they got sexual, and how ridiculous it all became, sometimes just for a laugh, I'd pretend to be both characters. She just sat there on the bed, she was only stuck there without knowing what to do. I was a disgusting child and I touched myself and she talked and I acted like the characters were doing it, and we talked and then we laughed. So when people say that they were afraid their parents might catch them masturbating, it's clear that not all people are from this planet. That's all I'm saying. That's all.

Strauss gently shakes his head. "To use one of your phrases, 'there really aren't words' to describe how misguided your family was. There really aren't." Sort of a smile, sort of sad. I don't even need pity at this point. I just want it all out there. I want it all cut out of me once and for all. "But for you to think it was *your* doing, that's equally incredible. That you played those games for you. That none of what you did was for her..." You're wrong. I'm sorry. For crying out loud, leave me something. I almost want to buy razor blades again. Or tacks. Any nice sharp point. Shopping for them can even be fun.

Cutting is a bit of a Rorschach Test - not for the *patient,* but reactions to it do tell a lot about one's family and friends.

Now that I've "confessed" the habit to Casey, I watch her glance at my arms and legs when she thinks I'm not looking. I don't do it anymore, babe. Honestly. Only scars are left. She says it's not so awful, promises it certainly doesn't affect the way she feels about me as her friend, and yes, I believe that and am grateful. What she doesn't say is that she simply doesn't get it. In fact, she claims it sort of makes *sense,* if viewed as something done out of the need to feel. As if I got numb and cut to bring back sensation. As if the numbness is some neurological event and my odd solution is nothing but a poor attempt to feel normal. And yes, there's some truth to that. But it leaves out one thing, dear sweet Casey. Leaves out all that emotion. The rage. My *pleasure* in the violence. It also leaves out choice. My decision to inflict self-injury was always a conscious intentional act. And the satisfaction from same. Casey's theory (much like her own self-image) leaves out every ounce of aggression.

Cleo, of course, just pretended the whole thing never happened. I was maybe kinda accident-prone. Bumped into things, like razor blades. *So* clumsy that I kept leaning against the tips of scissors. Amazing I could even walk. Cleo's little theory omits Reality - like her approach to life.

So the Strauss Lens for viewing this delicate little subject has been fascinating. At first he said the general things, I suppose. That it's not a good way to express. That he will not feel responsible if I hurt myself, it's my choice. That I can *tell* him things, instead of show him. Covering his bases. Or his ass.

But he's actually started asking questions like he wanted to understand. We look at it head on these days, my *pleasure* in the cuts. He's even said he can tell that I'm not ashamed of my scars, but instead seem proud of them. The man is much stronger than I would've ever guessed.

(Just *what if*, Cleo, what if you were wrong about people? This man, this doctor who I was only supposed to use, to manipulate for my meds…what if in spite of it all, I came to love him in a way – and he didn't destroy me?)

Watching you in sessions lately, your gestures, your hands. There's usually a cup of coffee nearby and I like noticing when you choose to sip. Need a little break? Fulfillment? Reaching for the Breast? Stifling your urge to say something? Or yeah, maybe, of course, just thirsty.

What does a woman want? Freud asked. And no one had an answer.

Every day I hear us, (NOT in the crazy way)…but in my thinking, our words, your words are becoming part of me. Part of my own mind. The other day you said that at this point in knowing each other, there's a part in *both* our brains that's "wired" for the way we are together. We see each other and immediately turn to that channel of relating. As if we're an Us. I suppose we actually are.

And when I'm alone, those things you've said are still around. Both the ones I cherish, and the ones I especially hate.

•   "You wear your pain like an emblem – that you are the Worst. That's the grandiosity. You get to be all alone with your pain and say no one understands. Just like you felt at home. To not see yourself as a victim – you'd have to give up the revenge against your grandmother – who is dead."

I walk down a street and feel surges of emotion. Remembering some conversation, I reel myself back in. They're only thoughts. My thoughts. From inside.

•   "If I look away from you for a *second*, and if you're already feeling rejected, then you'll take it as a sign I don't want to be here with you. You use reality to prove how you already feel. So your emotional state literally affects your reality. *Selective* perception and *selective* memories to give "evidence" to how you're feeling."

Still the existentialist, I challenge who I am, or might be. And others, those players in my life, extras mostly, some co-stars. How can I know what's real in what I see? Their faces are others from my past, and my own in their eyes reflect back people they've know before they knew me. We are strangers, all of us. And more familiar in delusion than we ever dreamed. And just perhaps, we all only see what we expect to see.

• "It was so hard for you to accept your mother and uncle knocking at the door when you were alone with Cleo. And that she also had strong feelings for her son and daughter...so much so that you had to block it out...to believe it wasn't even true. You still have to be the favorite all the time – and if you're not, you feel totally unwanted."

I am an adolescent whose hormones have just kicked in. The power of having a human body is enough in itself to require medication.

• "Connor has been the embodiment of your sexual, aggressive, wild self...the mind does not split in half, it doesn't work that way contrary to what some people may think. You've had your sexual feelings all by yourself, in the privacy of your own mind...you embalmed part of yourself where your mother and grandmother couldn't reach. But you can live with those feelings now. It's not as dangerous out here as ya thought..."

Last year at this time, I remember making one of my bolder suggestions.

"I think maybe I need to be in a hospital."

"Boy, now *there's* a good idea...." Of course you'd say that. "I'm sorry. But my opinion is that it's not a good thought."

"I might need it. That's possible. I won't if you don't want me to..."

"Look, if you'd choose to go into a hospital, it wouldn't change anything here. When ya got out, I'd be right here for us to keep working. But I am not going to encourage it, and I am certainly not going to put you in one!"

"Some people need to be taken care of that way...don't you help people make that kind of decision?"

"We're talking about you. And for you, no. Bad idea. Totally up to you to decide that for yourself." I'm so out of control and I feel like you think I'm only pretending. Tears like falling rain. I've gotten in farther and deeper, and it is no game. "You'd be in a hospital room still telling me I don't understand how bad off you really are. It's a vendetta against your grandmother. And you lost. She'll never have to face how hard it all was for you. The battle is over. You lost that one."

Words you've said over and over sound louder these days. Clearer. Things take a while to get heard.

"Children will do anything to win love. And one of the hardest things for the survivor of incest is the memory of the *arousal*. How awful it was, how odd it was...there's lots of sympathy for those. But also how *stimulating*, how *satisfying*...you weren't hurt or frightened by your grandmother. You hated it and loved it. Part of you wanted that attention to go on forever." It's so much easier to hate. "Two sets of feelings, usually many more than two..."

"This relationship between us here endures. The connectedness, the affectionate part holds us together through the times you feel angry at me. Relationships are much more durable than you ever believed. And even with your grandmother, you probably gave much more than you had to. She still loved her children even though they weren't as compliant as you. It probably wasn't as fragile in that house as you thought."

My relationship with Mary Jane *didn't* survive, you see. I started to hate her and I couldn't understand and I loved when I loved so so hard and she made me sick and I made her crazy and it was too much. And I just wrote her off. Cleo was enough for anyone. I had love. Besides, Cleo was perfect (at least once I finished with her in my mind).

Adore my grandmother.

Despise my mother.

Worship Casey.

Con everyone else.

Do what's necessary.

Wear a mask every day.

Doesn't matter, it's not really me.

What a lovely, tidy world it can be.

"You've tried to seduce people in, then walk away. Try to be what someone else wants, then instantly shut off, saying they mean nothing to you. Very sadistic."

"Your grandmother was *terrified* of her feelings. She used smoothing things out with the rest of you as a way of avoiding her own thoughts. I don't think you really *get* that. And you fantasize about doing that here – with me. Of one day just not coming back, or getting so sick that you end up dead, or in a psychotic state, hospitalized somewhere...and I would realize I never really knew you. Never understood. There's an incredible amount of sadism there."

"I think sometimes you hold onto a fantasy that you and I could go off together." Trust me, this silence is no game. "It's not ever going to happen that we have a sexual relationship. Won't happen. And it doesn't help you to think it could..."

"A sexual encounter with me would be incest. The worst possible thing that could happen to you. A violation of the relationship we do have, destroy you and destroy me, my career. It's one of the hardest things in treating incest survivors, they'll keep trying to provoke a violation from a caretaker...keep trying to repeat the trauma. And if it is repeated, the outcome is tragic."

"I only like the fantasy, that's all. I don't expect it to come true for god's sake!"

"Are ya sure about that?" It's gotten too dark today, that damn Daylight Savings Time and all. They give ya extra sunlight – and then just take it away. "I don't know how to say this to you in a way you can hear, without making you feel rejected, because I am not rejecting you. Not at all. But you do need to hear the reality of it. You need to be able to hear 'no.' You didn't have to hear that from Cleo." I listen. There's just little left to say. "By the way, this relationship here between us – its not fair. Not at all. It's not equal, and that's *just not fair* - but that's still the way it is."

I see of course. Of course you're right. And its all in my mind, the transference the games. I look at you and see someone else. I understand. I'm here because I'm crazy, not stupid.

It's not you, I want. For god's sake, I see that. Please don't think I'm *that* pathetic.

"Hi, Dr. Strauss? It's Janine. If you have any extra time, I was hoping to make an extra appointment..." It's our code. What I want to say is just *please call me back. I'm feeling crazy and I'm scared and I need you and I know I can't really need you because no one can say anything to keep someone else sane, but I miss you and to hear you talk for a minute, see I won't keep you long, but I hate that I do this, and hate that I'm asking but you don't seem to hate me, and you do understand. Please call me. Please. I need you, and that thought alone is so strange, and so "not me" I just don't understand who I am anymore. I need you. I do. God help us. Please call.*

The me who walked down the halls at work and admired the beauty, delighted in the image...well, she's gone home. Gone and forgotten. I despise every face I see from nine to five. Little pockets of conversations throughout the firm, the same words, different faces. He did me wrong. Doesn't understand how hard I work. I'm not appreciated. She stole my thunder. He did, she said. Poor me. Free for lunch?

The walls move. You sit there and whine about nothing, and I watch Reality shift across your faces. Forget it. Nothing new under the sun. My litany is just as old and tired as yours. I hear it. I see it. We'll all unbearable, but we can stand the smell from our own shit. It's just a fact.

I hate them looking at me, staring into my face. What the fuck do their eyes *want*? I'm not like you, yes, we all know. Leave me alone. Stop making me swallow. I didn't even want to suck.

Can't explain how it all happened, but I started getting angry and couldn't really stop. Then I went into the partners' bathroom and ripped off my pantyhose and shoved them into the toilet and flushed.

Stuff happens, you know. Stuff happens.

What I'd actually like to do is masturbate at my desk. Forget everything I see, and hear, and go off into my own mind and reach under my skirt and up my thigh and just take a little break.

Everyone's still talking about the overflowing toilet and those stockings. Well, people have to talk about something.

No, I did not put on another pair of hose. I walked around all day bare-legged, daring the bastards to see. Doubt if they did. It couldn't after all be one of their own.

Tuesday 3:30 Extra appointment, although now I'm feeling okay.

The re-release of *Belle du Jour*. Saw it again last Sunday. Twenty-something years ago that movie actually made me feel like I was not the only person like me in the world. It worried Mary Jane when she saw it. She was "concerned" about the stuff she didn't understand. I didn't have it in me to explain.

At least now Strauss will tell me when he's seen a certain film. Sometimes a cigar is only hoping to talk with a friend.

"Did ya see get around to seeing *Belle du Jour* again?" (It should be psychiatric required viewing. And today, we talk about her, that masochistic woman who can't resist pain. More than pain, she's driven by degradation. The beauty of Catherine Deneuve unable to enjoy itself without a crash into the dirt.

162

"And along with the literal sado-masochism," Strauss adds. "there's also her *martyrdom* in the fantasies about the crippled husband..."

"You're right," I love this. "She gives up everything to take care of him round the clock."

"Not a sacrifice out of love, though..."

"No, no, of course not. Just more of the same self-torment."

"Her guilt, right?"

"Maybe, but it's a dream sequence, remember. Less guilt, I think, than she's developed a more *sophisticated* masochism. Socially acceptable submission. Getting off in plain sight."

"That's interesting. But *is* it a dream – or more of her fantasies? That's not made clear..."

Talking. Ideas and words and talking. How did that alone become important?

The only way she enjoyed sex was to be with men who debased her, either through games and acts, or because they were repulsive to her sight.

Pleasure over the humiliation of feeling pleasure at all.

To find a kind man who loves you...well. Well, wouldn't that just ruin everything.

The men at Lara's didn't want their fantasies to come true. They weren't looking for real pain or subjugation in their lives. They wanted to simply get off, and they knew what it took.

The split between reality and fantasy is not one of degree. They are two separate worlds and the joys in one can be hell in the other. Today is not only talking. The Fights are on at ten.

"For you to maybe try to bring some of your hidden life out into the light of the real world.."

Oh, ya still don't get it! "Look, if you want to just *stay* in your cave, after all this work you've done here, just draw circles around yourself and keep the world out, that's up to you. I'm not going to agree with you though."   Could we have a tad less judgment there, doctor?!

Some things get *lost* if they actually happen. I suppose. Like if I were with you, just for example's sake, if we were lovers, if I wanted that, everything would change. My body might respond to your touch without recoiling, and my mind (already half-seduced) would delight in you delighting in me. That ain't the sex I've known in my head, sweetie pie. If I was aroused from our gazes, from the friendly dominance game of wit...if I could feel your hands move up my body...this honest to god, and no bullshit allowed...would...not...be...*me*.

When Casey goes from bad to worse, when she finds herself looking for Prozac along with half of New York, when now she finally decides oh, she's the screwed-up one, all I want is to turn my back. And I don't. We came into this together, and maybe she's where I belong.

"But you don't have to offer more than you can really do..." Strauss tries to keep tabs on just how far I've got the nerve to backslide.

"I know." No nod though. No lies. "She needs me, see..."

"It does not help her. *Ask* yourself if you honestly think what you do is good for her..."   Oh, that is the unspeakable part. Sometimes I just don't care if it helps or not.

Cleo always thought that the worst thing she ever did was leave Mama. Not that the lady was lonely, for Cleo was one of ten children. Her Papa worked in a tobacco field and when his wife announced (every year or so) that there was going to be a new addition, he just laughed and said, "okay, I guess there's room for one more."   Cleo made them sound like The Waltons, people whose happiness depended on nothing but air, a family whose love alone could provide a good night's sleep. When Cleo met Rankin at the telephone company where she worked as an operator, she was flattered she always said, so proud to think that this nice man liked her, and then loved her and wanted to make her his wife. Rankin was transferred out of the state right after the vows and it never occurred to poor Cleo that leaving home to marry meant she might have to leave home.

"We took a train," she told the story and I hated it more every time. Her eyes were sad in a way that wasn't Cleo. "That is such a mournful sound, a train whistle. We went too fast, see, I'd never been on a train before. I wouldn't have taken one if I'd known they took off that fast." Tell me about the time you and your sisters raised that Billy goat and he tried to sleep in your bed. Please Cleo, stop feeling sad. Nothing lasts, it's no one's fault. I'm sorry you were sad.

Some people feel too much. There isn't a category in the DSM for that one. For hearts that break too easily and sights that soar too high. There are drugs for mania, but they like to call it a delusional state that is corrected (reality-fied) by a combo of chems. There are people though who are well aware of what is real and how the world works and what living is like. And they just can't take it, can't not feel it, get no break from the love and the pain. They are the people who wake up from dreams so powerful that they're afraid to sleep again. To feel is a gift, but to feel too much... We're the drama queens, I guess, those princes of passion. Call us over-reactive. It's okay. Your words will fade.

"It's not feeling too *much* that causes the trouble." Strauss says. "It's the trying *not* to feel." Dissociation can result when someone is traumatized, but it can also happen as a result of trying not to feel. "Careful there, it doesn't '*happen*.'" I know. It's something I do. "Not to place blame..." I know. To see that I can stop.

I can't tell if he's curing me or controlling me. Or if there's any difference between the two.

What the hell have I done, taking in a dog? I worry about him every time I'm out of the house. It makes my chest literally ache to imagine he's lonely or scared. This gold and white hairy thing has too much power these days. I wasn't strong enough to have a dog.

For the first time I refuse to rescue Casey. "I don't want to be rescued!" she insists. I know. But you also don't want to take care of yourself.

I am not who I was.
We were right to be scared.

Some cars run best on their own.

I buy a large cloth net bag to carry Pugsley. On Saturday mornings I like to head to the bookstore and well, it's close to the Park and life is short and that grass is so tall.

"Worry accomplishes nothing. Do what you can to have things be good, and then don't worry." -- The Unabridged Annals of Cleo. (What d'ya know? Sometimes she got it right).

"That's an especially hard part of this," Strauss says with a nod. "To decide for yourself what to keep and what to discard. Easy to believe it all, or discount it all. Extremes. Harder to sift through, keep the good. It's part of growing up." Oh, that was *never* part of my plan.

I let them do so much more to me than I wanted. At Lara's. At the firm. At home. At Casey's. As if I couldn't say no, but I could have. These were not bad people, but at their hands...what I have done.

"You torture your*self* – in other people's names." And they never know. "And they have no idea what's behind your smile." The men at Lara's never knew. "Neither did your grandmother." But she should have. People should be able to tell... "No one can read your mind..."

It's a dance, the way we talk lately. Real. And quick. As fast as wit, but without needing to laugh. An actual mental connection with *words*. Inside each other. With no one pretending. I wonder sometimes if this is what other people are used to. When they talk of feeling close, is it this?

Words.
As something good?

The power of speech was never more evident that at Lara's. Certain phrases, words, the fetish sentence…a whipping, a foot. Her shoes. The skirt. Being spanked. Getting hard. Naughty boys. The saying of it had more power than action. And with my memory for detail, and acting background, with the simplest of scripts I could take a client on a roller coaster ride of his own body. Up and higher and higher and then…

Words, key words, like the flick of a tongue across the softest point of your flesh, sudden and cool, again and again. You wait for it, and nothing. You beg and still none. Then a hint, the shadow of your favorite word, a tease…with dripping lips a rush of air and you know its coming, the blink of an eye, the smile of an eye, we play a while to remind you its safe, a stroke a strike but lightly and loving, it's coming we're coming and the word appears in the air. Given to you like a velvet-wrapped present, handed over on a silver tray.

Of course they loved me. I was the keeper of the word.

And to know someone's word is to own him.

The difference between the clients and Lara's and the people at my mid-town, corporate firm is negligible. Everyone likes to play "look Ma, no hands! See?! Ma!!!! Pay attention here!" And for whatever reason, they all seek me out when they're in the mood. Elaine rambles on about her triumphant Phoenix-esque surge to freedom since a recent divorce. How he held her down, how she didn't see her own self worth, how she's her own best friend now, what she told him last week and-wasn't-that-something-wasn't-I-great-to-say-that-see-how-amazing-I-am…

No, babe, I honestly don't. What I see is that you're still married and his opinion is paramount and you've changed your costumer but not the script. And yes, I understand your growth is important to you. I know all little kids like to show off their treasures that land in the toilet. Come see what I did! SEE! Yeah. I see. But what *you* can't see is that everyone is more interested in their own shit, spectacular sculpture though yours may be.

The saddest price for my harshness as Doctor Know-It-All pointed out, is that I assume everyone else is thinking like I am. They're as uninterested in me as I've been in them. They're all wearing masks similar to mine. All mocking behind my back. Of course, I don't like being around people. I assume they're just like me.

"Okay," my smiles were never broader than when I met a new client. Had to make him feel safe. Comfortable. Had to tame the potential predator. "What kind of fantasy did you have in mind for today?" We sat in chairs around a small table like two nice Londoners awaiting afternoon tea. He, of course, was buck naked which was a bit of scene stealer. The men were asked to strip prior to consulting about a fantasy; no cop would strip. Few places to hide a badge. The other women always wore sexy garb for the consultation part, dressed in black corsets, fish net stockings, or low-cut red blouses revealing lacey underwear. A few would enter in nurse's uniforms, or leather pants. Not me. I wore a plain black jersey dress, moderate heels and street make-up. Not knowing what the guy's particular fantasy was, I didn't want to prejudice the game. One man's obsession is another man's joke. Leather makes some people roll their eyes, the same people who'd pay hundreds of dollars to see the right pair of shoes. Bondage turns some guys' stomachs, maybe the same ones who live to cross-dress. Fantasy buffs are as condemning as the next fella of a fantasy that isn't their own. I wasn't about to prejudice the game by offering a sampling of what they might prefer not to taste. They know why they're there. It's all that matters.

The man in front of me was unusually nervous. He reaches for a large towel and holds it tightly on his lap. Shaking his head, drawing in a long breath, he looks almost pre-heart attack. Sure, many guys have a tough time saying what they want to do, kinda looking at the floor as much as me, talking in whispers, peppering their words with "do you think that's okay?" It's a fine line to walk, making them comfortable enough to communicate without patronizing them with "oh, there's nothing strange about that at all..." In fact, not only do they fully realize that a lot of what they're saying is peculiar, they enjoy it that way. Feeling perverse, dirty, can be part of the fun. "I'm pretty weird, aren't I?" had to be played very carefully.

"I can handle you" was a good response. You're safe with me, yes, I'll play, but no, I won't reassure you that you're not a bad boy. Very little navigating room and of course, my specialty.

They loved me. Strauss thinks that's one of my grandiose delusions, but he's wrong. I was the intelligent, psychologically-savvy mother they all wanted, pretty and sexy, but not a glamour-babe. Warm and tender, dramatic and insightful. They were safe in my arms, but my mind was one step ahead of them. They were ten years old and I was Mom with very special cookies. Of course. I was Cleo.

"So you want to do a dominance fantasy?" I finally got that much out of the nervous guy. "What kind?"

"Regular dominance I guess." Well, no. There's no such thing. Mistress/slave games? Then I'll dress in a garter belt, leather dress and four-inch heels. We'll put you in light bondage, cuffs and chains tied comfortably around your ankles and wrists, affixing you to wooden posts at the end of a bed. I'll carry a whip or cat-o-nine tails neither of which I'll use at all unless we've discussed it. Most of the men didn't want pain, they wanted theater. My whip lightly touching their legs, my words taunting and mocking, my postures haughty and tempting. Tell me you adore me. Again. Again. Tell me how worthless you are. Again. Now stop. Close your eyes. You don't even deserve the privilege of looking at me. The whip cracks hard on the floor. Kiss it. Kiss the leather, boy. Impress me. You're boring me, boy. Careful. You don't want to do that.

Many preferred more realistic roles like teacher and student, notebooks and rulers and chalk boards surrounding us. Stand in front of the class, young man. Tell everyone what you were doing

*underneath your desk. Show us, little boy. Show the whole class
what you were doing. The men were not very good actors, they
mumbled many of their words, giving themselves just enough real
interaction to make the mental trip worthwhile, mostly holding it
all alone in the privacy of their own minds. I played my parts to
the hilt, never dropping character, never wavering. They'd take
what they needed, checking in with me, tuning back out. I was the
Reality they borrowed from to feed the thoughts no one would ever
touch. I was a waking dream for them, tempting them out of their
trancelike concentration, bantering about in the real room with
real words a hint of the play that lived in their minds. Then they'd
retreat, in and out throughout a session, away from me again, and
I kept going as if we were still together. Lost in his own mind, I
was out here when he needed me. Rapprochement, little toddler.
Wander as ya like, mom will be right here under this pretty oak
tree. Always watching. Ready to wave or rave at her precious
little man.*

*The bundle of nerves in front of me had grown edgier, not
calmer. "Look," I said, losing patience. "You can just tell me
what you'd like to do. There are many different kinds of
dominance games. I need to know your particular fantasies.."*

*"It's all so sick. Don't you really think so?" His face a
variety of reds, and still no eye contact. "I mean, I'm just
disgusting..." If I'd been new to the business, my heart might have
gone out to that guy. Poor schmuck, so hard on himself. But I
knew better. "I'm sorry," he said.*

You're right, Dr. Strauss. It can be a dead give away.

*After another ten minutes of hemming and hawing and
intense self-deprecation, Lara joined us to find out what was
taking so long. I welcomed the break for freedom, shook my head
at her in a way he couldn't see, and left the room. She stayed with
him for quite a while, then came downstairs saying he was going
to think about it a little more.*

"He'll be leaving in a few minutes," I summed up.

"No, I think I got him calmed down."

"Bet five?" *There were all kinds of way to make money there. But Lara knew better than to ever bet against me, and shortly the guy came walking down the stairs, fully dressed.*

"I'll come back some other time. I'm so sorry.." We opened the door and both shook our heads.

"Wanna go upstairs and clean up?" I asked. Then she seemed to get it. That guy had acted out his fantasy after all. He wasn't hampered by his humiliation, he'd been hiding an erection beneath that towel. Self-torture, self-ridicule. And we'd just sat there while he said all the key lines himself. When he was sufficiently worked up, he'd come. And gone.

Take away some people's embarrassment and their fantasies would dissolve. Often the arousal *is* the shame.

So Doctor, when you've said that oh, there's just nothing to be embarrassed about. I can tell ya anything. It's okay. Maybe I wasn't so caught in my own trap after all.

"Is that what you want for yourself? To keep having the same fantasies over and over? To keep playing out the same scripts..."

Do you have the slightest clue that sometimes as I sit here in your soft leather chair, as I lean back and stretch my legs...as I snuggle into its arms and press against its hide...and I tell you things that are so hard to say...and you ask me questions that are deliciously painful...and I sigh, and I look away, and you ask what I'm thinking, and I avoid, and resist, and try harder and again you ask if I'm okay...and when least expecting it, you go for the kill...and I reply and we stare and your eyes hold me like strong hands on soft velvet...and it's the first time in my life that I've ever lost control with someone else.

The truth about all that gets told over a payphone. Into your machine, that delicious part of you that can't talk back. All ears. Still you. But with a few extra miles between us. "I feel aroused by it, do you hear me?! The hard part of talking – it's also pleasure. The shame is part of the gain...and I try to get rid of it and I don't want to ever lose it. And I hate being that way, and it's more me than anything else... no way out. I suppose. I'll never change."

"As much as you hated your grandmother coming too close, your mother coming too close, *exactly that much* you also wanted them even closer…"

It's a Brain of opposites, this human organ. "Conflicts." Ordinary human conflicts.

Reality.

There are some things one just flat out wants to get to keep.

Don't take it all. Please.

I'll play in the real light. But leave me a little shadow for my own.

Newer thoughts that aren't familiar at all. Symptom-free. For days on end, I can think whatever I want, no… more serious than that – I can think whatever comes into mind. For the first time in my life, I'm not living every minute as guardian of my mind's gate. When I tell him, he nods. And that's all. My god, we should be celebrating!

"You somehow don't seem satisfied." I offer.

"*I* don't?" he laughs.

Well, one of us doesn't. You know those tricky pronouns.

There is a wonderfully caustic term called "flight into health" that describes what happens when a patient seems to improve all at once, usually early in the therapy process. Lacking any actual growth or change, the patient's symptoms just vanish and that marks a decision to walk away from treatment. *Well, hey, I'm okay now. Thanks much. Buh, bye.* But it's one more defense. Unwilling to face the intensity of the process to come, the mind calls off the troops and surrenders, as if to say *okay, UNCLE! See, nasty symptoms all gone. Now get away from that damn doctor.* It happens when the patient is scared to go deeper. It happens.

For the past six months, I've done remarkably well at staying out of Casey's dramas, enduring not as savior, but merely as friend. Not-mom. She watches me change and I imagine that

172

she's come to fear me. It comes out in our talks, over coffee, on bus rides. At lunches I no longer pay for. "It's okay," she says when the bill comes. "For god's sake, I can treat *you* once in a while..." As if it's ever been about money. I've never paid for anything with resentment, pal. All I ever did was what I thought was needed.

And when I brag to Strauss about my new autonomy I feel like some magazine success story. *Co-dependent Fully Recovered.* No longer needing someone else to need me. What I fail to say is how much I resent her lately for refusing to see what she does. Casey's crime is that she's stayed the same. And if I hate her for that, then it's clear I'm no healthier at all. The unmitigated gall in me to turn against *anyone* for being themselves.

If you were a better doctor, you would've helped me fix her.

And in that name of Rightness people wave wands over somebody else's freedom, casting spells to enhance - against mortal wills. As if I know what's best. Playing god. Being Cleo. Yes, of course I fucking see it. That doesn't mean it goes away.

Mostly I miss the way I used to *think* of Casey. Revisions have taken away every drop of solace.

Warm eyes, the good mother in her face. That laugh.

See, I was the sick one, always and only. "Mother" was perfect and would live till the end of Time.

And in that, my treatment has touched the untouchable, I want to tell him. You've made me see too much, and now in the name of medical health I'm expected to thank you? And then...yes, and then...I'll just be expected to walk away. From you. From us. From the only man I've ever wanted to love.

"So if I've taken Casey away, I'd better damn well be ready to replace her..." He does seem to see it. Then where is his guilt?

Monday 6 p.m.

"Let's talk about where you might want to go from here…" he says. The clock has never ticked louder. The session is always ending.

I'm quitting my job, that much is certain. Already written the resignation letter.

"Before you have something else?" he asks with that subtle worry. He says. He asks. We're only going in circles again. I'm sure he wants me gone. See, doctors have unconscious minds, too. On some level, he's gotta know I won't be able to stay well, and how tempting it must be to have me terminate while things look hopeful.

Reality. That much-hated theme that's pervaded our talks for a month.

"You can't use treatment to create more fantasies…" he advised. You mother fucking son-of-a-bitch.

You say I can tell you everything, but luckily I've maintained at least a little common sense. You'll never hear the most dangerous fantasies, babe. Not the really sordid ones about you and me and the Sunday Times. There are bagels involved, and cream cheese and those cranberry muffins they sell a few blocks away. Strong coffee and a thick fluffy comforter are props, and the set is a bedroom with colors like the ones in your rug. We can read together in the same room, the same bed, and touch and laugh and still stay separate. You take a sip of coffee and start reading out loud to me from the Book Review, in your most actorly voice, and when I kiss your hand, you shove the papers to the floor.

Thursday 5:45 p.m. Late as usual.

"Right," he says quickly. "As usual. But tonight for some particular reason, it's bothering you…"

"Maybe I'm just getting braver in telling you so."

A session of pouting. Of blame. No hourly rate too high for deep satisfaction.

"Your anger was projected *out* – onto *me* – when you said I won't face how bad your pain has been," he buckles down for the serious interpretative stuff. "It's *you* who's been putting a mask on everyone else – one of your own face. And when you get furious and plead with me to *do something*.... I think you were angry at *you* for a very long time – for not looking, not seeing ...for not *doing* more...to help yourself..."

"Honey, please," begged Cleo. *" We don't want to upset the House."* Yeah. Unfortunately, we resided in a very sensitive piece of architecture – whatever you do, do not upset the House. And over time, I became it. As impenetrable, as impervious, as frozen in my past as the lop-sided white stucco with every shade taped tight.

Who would've expected the world to end on a Friday? Seems so cruel to be cheated out of a last weekend. But the call comes at 5:20 on a Friday in the spring. Beautiful and peaceful day. Should've been a clue.

After living there over fifteen years, Casey is being evicted. The marshal arrived with a team of movers. It seems they have papers, legal documents citing failure to pay rent, ignoring of warning notices. She got no such notice, she swears and cries. Certified letters left at a post office, never retrieved because never faced. So a seven room apartment is being moved by strangers, and she begs for my presence, for my calls to her other friends. As if I'd never met Strauss, as if time itself had never moved, I'm racing through my memory for names of would-be helpers and then racing my own body to her disposal. For both of us to finally be disposed and done with, it seems. We pack and negotiate for hours upon hours that lead into the night. When the sun rises on Saturday, she'll be in my apartment, the two of us sharing a studio and plans being made about how best to retrieve her things, to right this wrong, to fix this (one more) injustice just one more time. Of course it's not your fault, Casey. We'll get ya through this. It's no one's fault at all.

I know better.

I do.

And I know there's no way out.

"But why do *you* need to get involved in all this?"   I've no choice. "Of course, you do!" I know.

"I'm just letting her stay with me for one month. I've told her, been clear." And it's true.

He leans forward, elbows on knees. Familiar position over the years. Emphatic pose. We know each other through and through.

"Why now?" he asks.

"Because *now* is when she got evicted!" Jesus, doctor.

"But you've been ignoring her last few crises…."

I haven't had a real session in weeks. We talk only about this, about her. Again, I'm no longer center stage. "I'm talking about all this *for you*." He seems angry. Well, fuck man, who *isn't* these days?

The work took so long to build and it unravels so fast. A single thread pulls a sweater into pieces with one yank of the heart. "You're *not* doing this for her," he argues. "You know better than that." This time I honestly don't. This is my dearest friend and she has absolutely nowhere to turn, and in bad moments, I almost feel like the whole travesty is my fault anyway.

"Oh, you should've paid her rent?!" No. Not so simple. But I could've said *no* before now. For over a decade I played into her delusions about herself, about us. The two of us against the world. Those were years she should've been learning and strengthening, but I just used them up for one more quick fantasy session. Let's play, okay? You be you and I'll be Cleo and oh, we'll watch time stand still.

"It took two." His words sound like a concluding remark. Nothing is really getting in, and he can tell. It's bigger than all of us now. See, yesterday flew in as a night sandstorm and it's covering the village, no, *burying* the village...we really should conserve our air and not talk so much.

"This is *not about* Casey," he adds, and I realize his comments are far from ending. "Can you see that? I agree that the timing is prime, but she and her eviction are answering a need...and it's far from about her."

It's about us, you think. That eternal couple, wedded together twice a week, and annulled when apart. Consummated in mind only and contract only...in the eyes of a god neither believe in and united by Father Freud. Yes, I suppose all kings think everything is about themselves. But then you have so many wives.

In truth, what's wrong with being left a few fantasies? You've said it yourself - we humans need defenses in order to *not* go mad. Once I liked thinking we were gonna be famous - Casey the Oscar-winner and me, and it was not impossible no matter what anyone believes. It's right that I faced some myths about Cleo, granted, I'll give us that one. Better to have seen. But there are years more to go on this earth for me, doctor. Seasons to weather and places to be. I can travel *light*, but let's get a fucking grip. I need a jacket or two or I'll die in the cold!

"You'll die of exposure?" Good one. And I smile. But seeing isn't always believing. Knowing is not always best. "Don't let all the work you've done here..." he nearly pleads. But time's up. Casey can't afford to stay in New York, and plans are in high gear to move back to Texas where she went to school. Things are so much cheaper there, see. Cost of living. And all. It's still been hard on me to work, that daily pain of subservience and yes, oh, yes, even without symptoms it's hell. I wouldn't need to work full-time in there, could get by on maybe four days a week. And build a new life. A life without craziness. He knows how long it's been since I had any episode at all, and we knew treatment had to end sometime. "Don't do this..." I can't let myself look into his eyes anymore. The days when I thought he hated me were days where I *was* crazy. This man has come to care, but see Casey also cares and too many people care for me to be able to think. I would have been better off if no one had ever loved me at all.

Then he asks a painful question, one I'll carry in my heart forever. "Do you have any ideas about why you've stopped trusting me?"

"That's not true!" It's one of the most painful things he's ever said. "Do you think if I trusted you more, I'd just do what you *say*?"

"Hardly." He is so serious today. We both are. "But over the years here, all the different feelings you've gone through...we could always talk."

"We *are* talking...."

"Even when you got very angry with me, there was enough trust between us..."

I trust you. With my heart, my life. My god in heaven, why are you trying to destroy us?

"You want to hurt someone when you think you need them." Now *that* is very true.

"What else do you want for *yourself* right now?" I don't know. "Let's talk about it then, explore...and see if you can find out..."

I've done it all, it seems at times. Performed here in New York (my god. In dearest heaven. Me. Center stage.) "You've performed a little bit, yes..." Maybe it was enough. In a perfect world, I would've tried to be the star. Is that what you want to hear me say? "No right answers here..." I know. But there's truth in it, see. I am well aware that if I'd been willing to live myself instead of living through her... "Then why on earth would you think about going off with her again?!" It's different now. "No," his face is so serious. "It is exactly the same." *I'm* different now or don't you believe that either? All my work, all our remarkable achievements... it's night. Kinda late. Time to sleep.

Cleo, come lie in my arms.

As Sheherezade wove the most beautiful stories night after night, he was charmed. Even though she was fated to die, he couldn't make himself order it as night after night, he looked more forward to the newest tale. She talked of people and families and love and loss until his heart was captivated. He was changed as he listened. As we all are when we listen right. The King fell in love, not with her tales, but with her. And soon it was the girl herself he looked forward to, and at the end of days, she was met not with death, but marriage. And it was his love, more than her words, that saved her.

Some children never have to hear 'no.'

Thursday 6:00 p.m.

It's our second to last session.

"I would not have believed it," I smile. "When I talked about being so sure, years ago, that I was literally going crazy. I knew I was right. Just knew it...that there was something wrong inside my brain."

"You're saying something very interesting there..." We're almost careful with each other again. Like newlyweds. Full circle.

"I'm thanking you. Sincerely. You knew I could get well and I had no faith at all..."

"Do ya even *need* me to point out what you're really saying here?" That beautiful smile should never look sad.

"That I was wrong then? And you were right?" A nod.

So I'm saying maybe I'm wrong again? And know it?

It's simply too late. My own situation has mirrored Casey's now, and I've got no job but behind in the rent. The only way out is out. Starting over.

And yes, okay, yes. I created it.

If I did stay, if I could, we'd wrap up treatment. It's going to end anyway and we both know. You've told me I can't stay in one place, can't freeze on one block in the Yellow Brick Road. Can't stop time to play with my fantasies forever - although I do wonder, why *not*? If I stayed, you'd try to make me see the man

179

behind your curtain. I do see him. I'm not *that* nuts. I know you're only a man.

But I also know me. The thoughts I've had of you, of us. There's nothing wrong with them, and they give me a pleasure I've never known.

Please let me keep a matchbook to remember I was here.

"So many feelings have awakened in you... and it must be terrifying..." Just one little fucking matchbook. Okay?

The one thing I withhold from Strauss is the *way* in which I'm moving. Not even telling my landlord, simply abandoning half of my stuff (well, the truck only has room for Casey's). We've packed her up, and I've sneaked in the only treasures of my own that matter, claiming I'll send for the rest once there's money. Oh, yeah, there's quite a lot we've planned to do when that Day Comes. I realize I'll never see the rest of my stuff again. Any of it. This is leaving par excellence.

In a way, I'm evicting myself; well, that's what he'd say. I know. I hear him whether he's around or not.

In the elevator, I morbidly wonder what will happen when they eventually turn off my electricity. A leaking refrigerator might alert someone that the girl has gone, I suppose. Ah, yes, new shame. But I was better. I *am* better. Maybe my symptoms are wreaking havoc in the world now instead of just in my mind.

The one thing I keep from Strauss is the way in which I'm leaving. Not telling the landlord, simply abandoning half of my stuff (well, the truck only has room for Casey's). We've packed her up, and I've sneaked in a few things of my own, claiming I'll send for the rest once there's money. There's been so much we've planned to do when that Day Comes. I realize I'll never see it again. Any of it. This is leaving par excellence.

Last minute packing and exhaustion – we're exiting in much the way we arrived, and certainly not in a way I'd do things alone.

180

But it almost feels right to be racing before some setting sun. There is never enough time in this life.

The day we leave, I write for hours in a journal. Those *will* be going with me, every word. I came home from every session and wrote in a spiral notebook. For over seven years, now twenty-three books, every day with Strauss has at least a page of insights gained, of fears and rages, of how he sat and what we wore. So many days, most in fact, where I wrote that *now* I understand...that *that* day's session put it all into focus. As if there is one encounter above others that makes the shift. Always knowing, well, that's me. Willing to admit there was a time I didn't, but that time is past, and now I see. Now I see. No more learning to fear. No more changes without my permission. Back in control. *That guy at the last gas station finally gave me decent directions and the next leg of our trip fell right into place. We're off and running now, babe. No one's lost anymore*, and we drive to that rapid sun.

At least it's not a matter of minutes, but hours, before we start doing it again, the two of us. Left alone and dependent on each other, we're soon wearing the costumes of our dead parents. Refusing to turn into who she wants me to be...she, Cleo. She, Casey. Hating her back for not seeing what she does, for not changing...she, Casey. She, every woman I've ever loved.

A war of domination over who can remold the loved one fastest and deepest. On the long trip, at different points we each ask "why are you *like* this?!" As if that's the better question.

Why are you going off with her to do it all again? Strauss hammered. He is hundreds of miles away, miles I put there. It's not that I need him, not like I've even *used* everything we learned anyway. No, not me, not one to be limited by growth. I've left the city I adore and opted for running. All the things I've wanted to do there, left wanting. Left dreams. And we put more miles between us... and me. Dear god in heaven, what have I done?

We move everything into the new apartment, and I watch Casey's hope start to build again. She can do this. At least, I want to believe that. Just make a new life here, and set some things right. I, however, cannot.

You can't go home again? No, actually ya can – but you might see it now for what it really is.

"I'm not staying." It's one of the hardest and easiest things I've ever said to her. She only looks disgusted, says I'm acting crazy again. Well, isn't that interesting that at least the word is finally out there. We talk into the night about how, yes, the trip was stressful and change is hard. So is staying the same, my dearest friend. It's gotten harder than it ever was. In the end it's daybreak, always time for her to consider bedtime. And she wishes me well, this genuinely wonderful woman. I love her. Regardless. Almost more now in a way. Then she tosses in that I'm making a huge mistake. Things are impossible in New York, and look at all the trouble I've had working nine to five...why would I give up this chance for an easier life...and hey, I've already gotten what I can out of therapy...

When she finally goes for a long bath, I call his machine and start begging for my old appointment time. I'll need to borrow some cash (from somewhere, not here) and on and on goes the drama. But I've been to the edge of the world and not quite fallen off. Again.

That night I re-read every word from those journals. It's like a series of images at the end of a movie, re-telling its story, folding over one another to draw a lyrical memory and the illusion, of course – that it was all clearly leading to this Present. Things appear *destined* in reverse order, as if it's all part of a plan, the way every event came to pass. In truth, there *is* no sense, and retrospect nothing but a liar. Sure, I understand my past. But I'm still clueless in Now.

Do you have any ideas about why you've stopped trusting me?

There is a possibility you won't let me back in. And maybe you shouldn't. I've used us, tried to make a mockery of the work. You said to me once that you wouldn't let me destroy my treatment.

You lied.

It may have been a last-ditch effort to lose myself in her. Too scared to go forward, I made a race back to the womb in denial of both death *and* life. Stasis. Safety. Once and for all.

Nothing is forever. "Then why do *anything*?' he laughed once. "Why even make the bed?!" Yes, but *you* wouldn't take me. Take me away.

"Can you see me when I get back?" (and do you hear the tremble?) " I mean...do you still have my time available?" What you undoubtedly have is the power to destroy me in a single word.

"Of course." Words are warmth in my veins. You'll help me then... to finish the gamut? "Of *course*."

Pugsley walks back into his old apartment as if he's just been for a long walk. Never doubted me, huh, dog? Dumb animal.

I want to believe I've come back without secrets, having seen what they cost. That no matter what, we can still talk, and not turn against each other.

I never actually meant to leave you. I just meant to run away.

"Oh, I was supposed to have come *after* you?" He's a little guarded today. Even I can't blame him.

"You said I left because of us."

"Partly, yes..." we both keep careful watch. "Maybe mostly. What do *you* think?" I'm listening now. Tell me what you meant.

On a very rainy Thursday, I walk into your lobby with an angry thought. For the past three days I couldn't get this out of my head. You'll deny it, and you'll probably hate me. But the words are coming out of my mouth.

I see why I ran.

So help me, you are not exempt. You are going to hear this, and you'll understand even it means I finally destroy us.

Transference. "I am not your grandmother," you've said again and again. And that I put masks on your face (as I do on everyone's) to only see who I need to see. "Replaying things not fully remembered..." I see the technique and tricks of mind. And no, I'm not exempt either, not from games we humans play. But I've seen more in that golden-lit room with you, and I've seen what's *there*. It has not all been in my head.

"Before I left..." Part of me wants to stop before I say too much. "...the months before, the way we were talking... it's like you *blamed* me for having fantasies about you.."

Can you see how real this anger is?

"Hold on there. *Never* did I say that...."

I *need* to do this. All of it. Only listen.

I can barely breathe. A rage that makes blood freeze.

"You blamed me for not seeing you as you." He wants to argue the word "blame" but I watch him stop, and listen. As if he's heard. And maybe for the first time in any session, my eyes never leave him. "...you said I was trying to turn you into some fantasy character, that I *fantasized* life, and stayed only in my head..." The right words won't come out. I don't want to say all this in such a state. Wait with me. This needs to be said and it can't if I'm looking crazy. *I am not crazy.* And so help me, god... "I know I'm upset, but I also know what I'm saying, okay? *I'm not crazy!*"

"I know that." Slight smile. "I've always known that..."

I AM NOT THE ONLY ONE HERE.

I AM NOT THE ONLY ONE WITH *FEELINGS* IN THIS ROOM.

"It hasn't all been my doing," I'm gasping to breathe. *"Not all in my head.* The way you are with me, the way you've been. We got to know each other, and *you* changed, too. In the way you were with me. Showing me more of yourself. And yes, I know it was mostly that I could see you, when the smoke cleared and I saw you, not them...but you also didn't hide yourself, how you think, what you like. You enjoyed it too, the way we talk, about movies, and books. You *like* that I'm smart. I've seen you *compete* with me, I've seen it, I've watched your male fur go up if I make a literary reference, and then suddenly you're quoting poetry or talking mythology and making allusions to show off for *me!*" His face is serious, no nodding. No movement. Technique called up from the depths of memory I imagine. "It isn't fake, isn't technique. There is a part of you that *fits* with me, and yes, it may be technique to choose to *show* it, but it's *real.* The way you've smiled, that smug way if you've said something smart, and we *play* - you even *said* that we play. Don't tell me it's all transference! That I'm pretending you're someone else. It has not all been in my head! *I am not the only one with feelings in this room!"* He listens as closely as I've ever seen. And I can only wonder, how close is death? I believe everything I've said, but it was a mistake. It wasn't necessary to do this, it was...of course, it was. Maybe it was necessary to kill us off.

Leaning towards me, looking confident, warm. Please know it's not some trick, I want to reassure. I don't know why I did this. Please. "Is there a real relationship here between us?" He asks. "You *bet*." These expressions are as careful as the first day we met. And your eyes, so sincere. Okay, yes, yes, there's an "us." Let's leave it at that. It's okay.

"Okay," trying to smile. "I'm sorry to hit you with all this. Let's let it go..."

"Oh, no..." a little playful. But not very.

I've ruined us.

I've made him afraid.

"I think we should talk more about this" he's so so careful. "Keep going with your thoughts." When I let myself look at his face, and then oh, that precarious verb – when I let myself SEE... he actually seems okay with this. All I'm doing is *asking*, I'm not challenging, I know I sound like it, but it's just the way I sound…all I wanted to do was *ask*.

"I want to know if you're aware of it, too." I try to keep going. I've done it before, survived it before. In this room if nowhere else in the fucking world, I know I can keep going. "That's all. I'm asking if you even know that you sometimes flirt with me…"

Is there a class in psychiatry that teaches you guys how to keep your heads so still? No nod. No shake. No comment subliminal or otherwise. Not an inch of movement. It's really a remarkable skill. "I'm okay…" breath. Slowly. Calm. We can talk. Talk to me like a person, not a crazy girl, not a child. A grown woman. "But I need to ask. I don't even know why, but it's stays in my mind, the wondering and I get so goddamn furious. Not asking has become torture. And yes, of course, I know you may not tell me at all. I know that."

"Tell me again what it is you're asking." The two of us are not playing now. At least your face shows you know.

"That I haven't just made it all up." I feel my eyes glaring at him, and I don't hate, don't want to hate him. He hasn't done anything, but the anger underneath my voice is pounding. I hear it, I see how I must look. I don't even understand exactly what I'm accusing you of. "The way we can *be* with each other. Sometimes when I'm feeling okay, and we disagree…we *play* with each other here." Again, I can barely breathe. "We flirt. We *both* flirt. And I want to know if you're *aware* of it."

"I'll answer your question, okay? I will. But first I want to point something out – what an interesting way to put it – "am I *aware* of it". You're not doubting your sense of reality, not at all. You're asking me if *I'm* conscious …or if I'm hiding, if I'm deceiving myself…if I realize the way we can be with each other…and can I be aware of the satisfaction it gives *me*, too…" Yes. Yes!

Like Cleo…

"You're finally letting yourself wonder if she was aware at *all* of the pleasure *she* got…" Not possible. "in the bathroom." She just did what she did for me. We said, anyway.

"That's right," he jumps in. "That's what the two of you *said*."

"in the bathroom..."

"That's what she had to believe..."

"and bedroom...that she wanted to do all that. Couldn't see that she liked it, too."

"Right," he says gently. "That she was enjoying it, too."

"No, she couldn't let herself see that...so she did it all for me. So much as for me."

There's silence. And he lets me be. "I hate that, ya know."

"It must infuriate you. How could it not?"

"Beyond words." Through tears I half-smile. "But *you*..." I turn playful in the midst of the wreckage. "We were talking about *you*, doctor."

"Are ya gonna think I'm avoiding you if I ask *one more time* for this question?"

"You've said you get something out of this, what you do...that it's like a detective solving a mystery, a puzzle, yes. But here with me, sometimes there's been more. That sometimes there has been something flirtatious between us. Ego feelings. Male and female ... and from the way you seemed, from your eyes, you've enjoyed it, too."

"You're asking whether or not sometimes with you, probably with all my patients...are there ever sexual feelings in this room?"

Yes.

His expression is so strained. Clearly he doesn't really want to go there. But this is no trick, I want to promise. If I've ever been sure of anything in my entire life, it's that. I just want to know. No, I *do* know. I want to hear if you'll deny it.

An avalanche of sadness and joy. Seeing more than I really wanted. Some things never do change. Yes, Cleo. You got away with it. Without ever having to see.

"I'm not your grandmother," he says gently. "I'm not putting it all on you." I nod, and without warning, my tears start. "Is there sometimes a sexual crackling here between us? Yes."

Dear god in heaven.

187

"Do I enjoy the teasing that goes on with us? Of course I do." He says it so emphatically, not playful. No mixed messages, of course, I understand. Just the facts, sir. And that's fine.

All is fine if it's true.

" This is a professional relationship, yes. But we're also two human beings. And can't be a sterile laboratory, this room. Sex is a part of life, a wonderful part. Here in this room, it has to be a matter of degree, but...yes, of *course*, I see that you'd need to hear this. Yes, there have been moments of sexual teasing here – between us. That can even be useful, to see where you are in your treatment. But most importantly, I trust myself never to act on it."

I'm blown away.

His brow, deeply furrowed. Must be wondering now if saying so much was a huge mistake. It's okay, I want to say. You'll never know what you've done for me in this. I needed to hear it. Needed to ask. The asking was life and death.

"To know that I'm aware of it, right? That I'm aware of enjoying the playing that goes on here sometimes. Of *course* you needed to know that – because your grandmother enjoyed it, too. And *that*, you never knew."

And that I could never have asked.

All for me. She would do anything for me. Whatever I said, whatever I asked. For me.

"For both of you."

Playing horrible little games.

"No," he interrupts. "...not horrible, not evil. *Completely* inappropriate. Damaging. But not horrible."

Stuff I thought up. And made her do. "Stuff she enjoyed. Stuff she asked you to do..."

There was so much love. "I'm sure there was." So much. And that was ours, the love belonged to both of us... "*All* of it belonged to you both."

That you enjoy us. Banter back. Tease me back. I did not make it all up. It hasn't been only me with all the feelings in this room.

Not all in my head.

Not all in my mind.

Not all in me.

"Have I ever felt ripples of arousal here? Of course." Still a warm smile. Don't let this change us. Please don't be afraid of me. "And so have you."

"Yes, of course. Of course me." Of course both of us.

I am not crazy.

Look at that - out the window. The world is still here.

Cleo never even loved her lover. That won't leave my mind. Was she doing it all for him? Even Mary Magdalene wasn't that much of a saint.

"Your grandmother was *terrified* of her own feelings, so she put them onto everyone else..." We lived in a covered pot, smoldering passions. Never known. "It was a hot house. All those emotions, that anger wasn't only in Otis. The sexual thoughts weren't only in your mother. It's amazing how controlled everyone managed to stay..." Cleo was very powerful. "She was very motivated."

Here's a gruesome little thought...I bet you don't know I could go right back there in an instant, right into the bathroom, right into the bed. I could play out Cathy and Heathcliff with her and not bat an eye..

"Of course you could."

My fantasies have changed. I haven't told you that, how much Connor's changed. How's that for growth? I stay the same, but my fantasy character grows up...

"Maybe *they* have been taking their cues from *us*." Fantasy borrowing from reality. What a concept.

Years ago, that night the call came, I knew before answering. Not one of those New Age coincidences. For months, I'd known Cleo was terribly sick. The last two weeks, she'd been in bed, not able to come to the phone, so I told Otis to say how much I love her, and would talk to her soon. We all acted like she'd be okay, of course. And we all knew. She always begged not to die in a hospital. Ninety-seven. Ya sorta have to grant that wish.

A few days earlier, Otis called to ask me if he should try to reach a doctor. He wondered aloud should he maybe call an ambulance if things got worse...but she wanted to be at home, she kept saying it and saying it, and they'd smile and sit together and watch TV. He held her hand and only napped when she did. He told me he'd do anything but didn't know what to do.

How cruel it would have been to strip away her control in the last moment. This woman who called every shot, who took care of us all in the strangest and most loving of ways, she had to die the way she chose. Anything else done in any name of caring would be sadism disguised in a bad wool coat. "Leave her there" I reassured. "She loves you so much, Otis. She trusts that you'll do what she needs."

When I heard his voice that last night, and knowing instantly that I'd never again hear *hers*, he cleared his throat and said "hello, Janine, this is your Uncle." He'd never called himself that. Maybe he needed to say the word "uncle" out loud.

She died at 12:07 a.m. and he was there, had been holding her hand. She'd been dozing on and off and took in a deep breath, and died. He'd stayed right there for over an hour, wanted to make sure she was gone. Not for himself, he added, but for her. In case she woke up, he wanted to still be holding her hand.

I'm filled with bitter envy for a moment. That it was him and not me. Not my hand.

Otis is strong. Who'd have ever believed that would be said?

I tried to cry. The other half of my soul dies, and I only tried to cry.

Don't ever leave me, please please please.

"I won't. I'll live to be a hundred and five." Ya almost made it. The tears are mine now. The missing. Longing for someone dead and gone.

What must he think of them, my wonderful terrible family? The rape we've conducted of their very souls could make De Sade look tame. Together in a quiet room with fading sunlight, day after day we've drawn, quartered and splattered the truths of three human beings, and then tossed them into graves – all in the name of saving me. Even their ghosts tried to leave quietly.

I love all three of them...those people we've ravaged. And today my heart literally aches.

"And they loved you. That is so clear..." The kindness is right. If its not too late, let's stay respectful. "Do you understand that for as peculiar as your upbringing was, and..." then that chuckle, gentle but head shaking for emphasis, "they were absolutely as odd as anyone I have ever heard of....but they did love you. *So much.* And you knew it. They showed you every day. That's really why, in spite of everything, you're okay. All three of them - they gave you the ability to love."

In my mind, the epitome of self-love is this tattoo on my arm.

Something physical that actually pleases. Done right on the body. "Why Madwomen Paint."

Like the "no" in my leg, but more. Strauss once said that when I carved "no" into my thigh, it became my first published work. To have that seen, to have it understood and not mocked or condemned. It was a turnaround of sorts, the day he said it.

That's how most of my changes have happened - from some moment of feeling genuinely understood. Seen. As if that was a green light for my Self to cross new streets. I wonder if I'd been holding on for so long to so many secret versions of me – all the while hoping to show them one day. Keeping them well intact, in case. In case anyone would ever be allowed to see. Select viewing of my tattoo available in the Spring.

And when Strauss first looked at that artwork on my upper arm, his expression was dear. It was nothing like his gazes at my cuts. Not even particularly doctorly. More amused.

Delighted, one could say (if one was inclined to such ravings).

Interested. With a clear desire to understand.

And with affection. It was in his eyes.

Cleo, what if…just what if…that's how this man has come to feel about *me*? Only asking, dearest heart, but what if you…please don't get upset….what if you were wrong? Maybe not everyone out here is phony or cold, just playing us as best they can. Merely for argument's sake (and I've gotten good at those), let's say that in the years I've spent with him, showing who I am, learning who that is, and seeing who *he* is…not just using or stealing or covering tracks … anyway, dear Heart, it was only a thought. And thoughts can't really hurt us after all.

When I was little, Otis liked taking me to the grocery store. We both rode on his bicycle with me sitting on the bar, leaning back against his chest. He had one arm around my waist, one on the handlebars, and when we needed to shift to a new gear, he's say "okay – Now!" And I'd slide the lever to give us more power. One day as we came out of the store with Otis carrying a big bag of potatoes, a man in the parking lot stared at us, and for a minute it was frightening. But the stranger smiled as we got closer and watched us as Otis unhooked his bike chain. "I'm sorry," the man said. "Didn't mean to intrude – I just have to see how you and your daughter are gonna do this!" and then he laughed. Otis smiled a little and we climbed on. He held the bag in his lap, kept one arm around me, and I leaned my shoulder back to press the groceries in place. "Okay now!" and we shifted into second. The man laughed again and waved.

We told the story when we got home, and Cleo laughed. Mary Jane was worried of course, wondering what that man really meant.

"What he said was that he wanted to see how my little girl and I were gonna do it!" Otis repeated. "I guess he *figured* I was her father… it didn't matter, ya know. I didn't bother saying I was her uncle. We'll never see him again." And we understood what he really meant.

My mother looked like a movie star. Everyone said so. And when she had a little child, she managed to get a job. Every day

192

she left the house at 5:20 in the morning and before she left, she wrote me a peculiar note. It was left on top of the TV set in the front room, and Cleo would get up early and read it to be sure it was okay. (To this day I shudder to imagine the ones that didn't make her censor's cut). One note in particular:

My darling Janine,

I had THE MOST wonderful dream last night! Of course you were in it, too. (It was more than a "dream" Janine, I KNOW YOU UNDERSTAND!!!!) I was talking to Ted Kennedy and he was in Heaven, and he told me all the dead movie stars were there, too. And they loved me! DO you believe it?! They all know how I prayed for them, he said, and he said that one day when I come there, but that will be a long way off, but one day I'll be the QUEEN! Now don't say anything, Janine. Don't please. But naturally they want you there, too. I said I Couldn't go without You, of course. And I know they'll Want Mama and Otis, Teddy said God didn't CARE if Otis was an agnostic. So everything will be wonderful!!! I love You, Mom.

Once in a very convoluted moment, I asked Strauss "Would I even be *treatable* by anybody but you?"

"Careful there," he sighed. "Don't idealize me. I might not survive the fall."

You survived it, Cleo. I used to call you a saint, and you'd laugh and deny it, but I know you loved me for saying so. Some people feel safe only when adored. No blame there, my queen, I well understand. But now we've torn apart childhood photographs and found very dark scrawlings underneath. We've read unedited versions of my memories, and you, dearest Cleo, oh, you did not emerge as any saint.

But there are untouchables, there are. Memories firm as iron, pure as gold, that never change. On Saturday morning, we sat on the bus together and laughed, both so excited about our private day. You whispered that you had a little extra to buy me that shoulder-strap purse like all the girls on TV were carrying. For hours we shopped and laughed, and we ate French fries at

Woolworth's and talked about everything in the entire world (or so it seemed). Then I told you to wait by yourself near the photo booth in front of the store, and I raced back to where they kept the silk flowers and picked out a rose. You loved that deep fuchsia pink and I'd seen one back there. That night it stood tall in a vase on the breakfast room table and it lit up your face as much as the room. We'd taken some pictures in that 50cent photo booth, two beaming faces tightly pressed into each other, as if the frame wasn't big enough to capture both of us. Too close, cheeks smashed together. The smell of your powder was a kiss on my face, but later we laughed at how silly we were to think there wasn't more room. When we put them on the table, Otis said we looked alike, and Mary Jane agreed, not showing at all if she minded. All she added was that we were both so very pretty. We were. There was nobody in this world I wanted to be with but you.

We had a lot of Saturdays. Nothing could ever dim them, or taint them. Strong and lasting as iron, soft and precious as gold. The alchemy of that one, dear Cleo, is no secret. It is, however, a kind of magic. Without question.

Monday 6 p.m.

I want to make some changes.

"Uh, oh…" Didn't see that one coming, doc? I'm not changing *you*. Chill. "You've been fighting with me for so long…"

"*I've* been fighting with *you*?!" he gasps.

"Okay, okay…but you do have strong opinions… and you said I should get out in the world, right? Well, I found a writers' group, through Mensa…and submitted some of my stuff. They're gonna let me know."

Never one for moderation, the next week, I walk in with a catalog from Columbia. Adult continuing education. Life-long learning, they call it. A class called The Philosophy of Physics may not be the most practical selection for a woman without a career, without a clue.. Still, it's the one I sign up for, and something is better. I don't even know what, but something is better.

"You really *are* exploring out here in the world...maybe to meet people with similar interests." Don't put a name to it. You'll ruin it. Something is better.

They say ya don't fully understand your parents till you have children of your own. One Puglsey, one proof. I'm making every single mistake with him that they made with me. He's spoiled, he's babied, he's overprotected. When he encounters a stranger, he emits a sound reminiscent of the Baskervilles. In my arms, he melts and lies calm as a cat. This little guy knows he's loved. Yes, Casey, my dog is a bit neurotic. He also laughs most of the time. (canine equivalent is lips open wide to the side, tongue exposed, eyes up...all that's missing is a "heh, heh.") Did I mention that he recognizes the names of his toys? If I say "go get Mousy" he can pick her out of a jumble of a dozen squeaky figures.... He kisses me awake if I try to oversleep. The amazing thing is not how much he loves me. No, that's not the amazing thing.

Thursday 5:30 p.m.

"I finally figured out why I hate waiting for you..." I start talking even before reaching my chair. He chuckles, but looks appropriate braced. "Well, I did have a lot of time out there today to formulate a theory..."

"All right, let's hear it."

"It's because you *know* I'll wait. Not every patient would. They might decide it's not acceptable and quit, go off to look for a therapist with a good watch..."

"Yes, you're on a roll today.." He just has the best smile.

"Anyway, it's like I'm left waiting in bed for you. I've primped and fluffed and I lie on the sheets and you know I'll be there - whenever you decide to waltz in."

"That it's a power play.."

"Yep..." The most frightened child in the world has grown up to be fearless.

"You may be right..." He nods slowly. "That it's a kind of exploitation?"

"You're so patient here with me, probably with everyone...maybe you get a little of your own back out there, making *us* wait...those of us you trust not to go search for another bed."

His eyebrows up, he doesn't really look so ready to attack. "Seriously, you may be right. I'll think more about it, that it could be a vying for power...But why *today*? Why would you make this discovery today?" And we're back onto me, but not at the cost of you hiding. A place to play with unexpected comments free to flow.

There is this man, just a guy, anyway, and he's part of the writers' group. I can't begin to tell you how reluctant I am to even bring this up...

"Of course you are." Strauss laughs. "You think I'm gonna force him on you!" Well, you will. Let's admit we've made some impressive progress here, babe. At least one of us can face Reality now.

"He's extremely smart...a physics teacher. And science fiction writer... I don't know. I'm really not in the mood to discuss it."

"Ya like him..." Did you not hear me? "I heard *all* of it..." Smiles. Are you jealous? That I might find another man I like besides you? "What's his name?" Oh, now wait a minute. I don't want you getting all attached...

"Jeffrey." We're friends. That's it. Okay? We joke around. Yes, he likes me, of course I can tell. He picks on me. Pulls my pigtails.

"You're flirting with each other." Yeah. Just wanted you to know.

It's fun, yes, must admit. See, mostly it reminds me of the old Jack and Connor games. Out in the world, that's what we were aiming for, doctor. Good god, who would've believed?

Anyway, what tickles me about this guy is that he's such a stuffy dresser. Not fair, I guess. He looks quite good, but the details and probably the *cost* of those shirts and ties... I must look like a bag lady to him.

"So all of you went away for the weekend?" Strauss with that rare approving grin. "Upstate?"

"Yeah, one of the writers had access to this large house..so we did our meeting up there. Pugs went along, of course. Anyway, Jeffrey. On the drive, he was making fun of what he calls my "Morticia" shirt, long black silk with frayed sleeves...he knows I'm interested in magic, the darker...elements."

"Very Addams Family?"

"Right. Then later when we were getting bedrooms assigned, he ended up following me...I think he wanted a room close to mine, and I'd already chosen one at the end of a hall...anyway, several of us passed it and he said to Nancy "okay, so this is where the séance will be held tonight?" That kind of stuff. Like I said, we pick on each other."

"You like this guy." Strauss nods with the comment. Urging?

"He's extremely smart, and yeah, I if I have to talk to *some*body, he's not bad..." Strauss laughs hard.

"My, what a wonderful compliment!"

I feel like I'm 13 years old.

I might try this. This guy. A couple of years ago, I remember flirting with a few guys and that of itself was an amazing feat. But if I was looking at all then, I was looking only for someone I could pretend was Strauss once the lights got dim. This Jeffrey is a different sort. Grown-up. Smart. *So* fucking smart. And in some ways, so goddamn normal.

Monday 6 p.m.

"Wanna hear something that makes no sense?" I ask. "My family, long buried...I miss them more now. Lately. Some days I *feel* their deaths... like they happened yesterday."

"Makes *perfect* sense..." he says quietly. "No need to mourn when the past is still right here in the present."

As if nothing is ever lost. Or out-grown. Carrying memory everywhere and calling it observation. "Literally," he adds. "as if it was happening Now."

With no need to look back. It stayed right beside me.

Blocking the view of anything else really here.

"As much as I used to want to forget them sometimes..." I confess.

"You also were terrified you might..."

"Yeah. The way I imagined you'd forget me. That you'd be completely untouched once I left. As if I'd never been here at all."

"That doesn't happen." He looks almost sorry for me again. "Now you can make it happen – by hiding away forever, from everyone, never letting another person see you..."

"Dying without anyone ever knowing I was here..."

"Right."

"If I let go for an instant, I'd vanish. Disintegrate. No one knew me and I existed only in my mind..."

"That's what you wanted. Well, part of you did."

"Total freedom, it felt like."

"No needs you couldn't meet all by yourself."

And it looked like such a good idea at the time.

Thursday 6 p.m.

"So have you gotten rid of poor Jeffrey yet?"

"No." No reaction. "Maybe I don't want to give you the satisfaction." With that he just looks confused.

"Why would that *please* me?"

"To think I'm so predictable..."

"Ah, so I'm in a no win situation here." I nod, not even trying to hide the pleasure. "Look, I am not about to declare *any* preference on this topic... You won't get away with saying you did or didn't pursue this for *me*!"

"Can we be serious a minute?"

"I was being *very* serious." That grin is way too smug. "But sure...what is you want to tell me?"

That Jeffrey asked me out, and as much fun as we're having with the flirtation, as much as I could honestly think of him as a friend....this is not somewhere I want to go.

"Only a friend?," he asks gently. "You're not attracted to him at all?" He's attracted to me, or so I imagine. I don't know. I do not know. But it's all getting ruined with his pushiness. "Because he asked you on a *date?*" Yes, I was expecting that chuckle.

It was the way he asked that scared me, I suppose. Calling on New Year's Eve from a party. It seems he'd been telling himself to work up the nerve to ask me before the end of the year. With about an hour to go, I get this zany phone call from a highly nervous man in a loud room. Just to go out and see what happens. Just maybe go ice skating this weekend. Ice skating and lunch? It's going to be cold but sunny, pretty skies. Thanks, a good weather report is always motivating.

I've been on maybe five dates in my life. And never because I actually wanted to go. I was a teenager and trying to do whatever I could to not look strange. Shop. Date. Smile. Primp. As if I'm of this world. I don't even remember their names, those boys who drove me to a movie, or a party, and tried to kiss me but hardly talked at all. I was pleasant enough (10 mg. Valium) and none of them knew there was a mad girl in their car. In fact, they were stunned when I didn't want to go again. I wasn't *scared*, and I'm not scared now. I'm just not *interested...* who the fuck knows? Whatever...

"Jeffrey knows a lot about you, right?...from the writing you've shared there." Yeah. That is without a doubt the only reason I'm even considering it. He's *read* about me, see. My life, my self. He's read some of this book.

"The appeal must be that I'm a freak. What a challenge, right?"

"Yep. That must be the reason he likes you." So there is no sympathy anywhere for this one. Not in this room, *that's* clear. And certainly not from Casey, the poor woman with a arm-length list of bad men. Cleo was so relieved that I didn't care about dating. Men are very dangerous if you don't know what you're doing. She went through it with Mary Jane, and how wonderful to be spared that hell with me...

*"The only man I really liked was Matt," Mary Jane said it only once. "He was Geneva's son..." Her cousin. Oh, yeah, that fits. Let's never go **too** far outside the family. "He was nice to me. Matt was a nice nice boy, but I didn't want to get married, you know. Never did want to settle down."*

"Did you and Matt have an affair?" I know, I know, but I am nothing if not morbid curiosity. Tears came into her eyes, and she looked away. Never mind, I want to say. Forget it, I don't even want to know. She suddenly seems so old, this Simone Signoret look-alike, lounging in a long, lavender jersey robe. Her body still posing like her pin-ups, It's automatic now, not conscious. It's just the way she is. Her eyes look at the window, which is, of course, closed tight beneath taped shades, but she keeps staring as if she can see right past it. The tears start falling, gently, easily. Not in that hysterical way we're all so numb to. "I don't think so," she finally says. "I just don't know if we ever really did it, or not..." She's not the kind of woman ya hug, my mother. So we sit there, and she keeps looking out to places she cannot see.

Anyway, doctor, he kissed me. Not on the first date, well, he wanted to, I think. But he said he wasn't sure, and oh, yes, I do like it that way. See, this guy *wants* me, Dr. Strauss. Who needs you?

(There are too many people in the room.)

But I *felt* it. Him. His mouth.

I let him kiss me. I wanted him to kiss me.

We stood in the park in the middle of the day, well, the light looks safest then. And we touched, our bodies and our mouths kind of reached. And it did not feel like a movie.

200

"Can you imagine how a parent would feel?" Strauss asks with the most tender look he's worn to date. "A father...can ya *imagine* how he'd feel if his daughter came in and told him about her first kiss? He'd be *warmed*...thinking his little girl is growing up..."

Cleo would have been so afraid. And Mary Jane would've reached for 100 mg of whatever we had in the medicine chest. Otis? Always a good reason for beer, and then he'd have rambled about the cruel men he'd known in his life... No, I doubt anyone there would have been particularly warmed.

"I do need to admit something...it's something you really do need to know..." I say nervously to Strauss a week later.

"Uh, oh. Is this is like a veil beneath a veil?"

"Okay, okay...I'll continue as if you're interested ..." he laughs. "But this is hard to say, for real. Jeffrey. The attraction and all. Yes, I am highly attracted to him. It's intense, okay? It is. But we're overlooking something, and I need to put it out there. This is not some healthy step, okay? I've known this, but hated to tell you. The reason I think I like him so much – it's for the wrong reasons. He reminds me of you. Do you *see* that?" He takes a sip of coffee. If I had more time, that one would be fun to explore. " I wouldn't have even gone out with him except for the way we related to each other, the teasing, the banter...it was like us. It's still transference. But now I'm transferring off of you!"

He smiles. "Sometimes that happens. Each time, a bit more removed."

"And you don't think that means I'm using him? Just one more game..."

"I wouldn't discount the relationship that fast. We all like who we like for *some* reason, from something in the past...that's just life."

"Are you serious?"

"Besides you just *like* sarcastic people," he laughs. "The aggression is right out there. Not hidden. No tricks." Well, that's certainly Jeffrey. Right out there. Remarkably secure. He did analysis years ago, in England - and that means a lot to me. We had kind of an argument a while back, about closeness, my fears...he was saying we should just take the whole thing easy, no

201

pressure, his thoughts, oh, lord…anyway, he ended with "Oh, I think for anyone who wants to be seriously involved with you, being successfully analyzed should be a *requirement*." And then we kissed.

Thursday 6 p.m.

"What if he wants to have sex with me?"

"Whoa! Do you really think he might want that?!!"

"Have I mentioned I'm looking for a new therapist?"

"Ah, what was *that* remark about? Besides your signature attitude…" No, no! Nothing. I was joking. "I know that. But telling me *today* that you're thinking about replacing me with somebody else. I'm wondering if the subject is jealousy?"

That you'd be jealous of Jeffrey? God, I wish you were.

But in truth, he's more than that, this man. More than an object.

Oh, yeah. More.

When he looks at me, I melt.

This man who has become every cliché.

And I'm not much more than a teenager dealing with her first love. Maybe he will be. Well, no. My *second*.

Okay, Mom, this one's for you – Jeffrey looks like Michael Caine, the way he was in *Educating Rita*. Intelligent, reserved, with the most beautiful quick-silver smile.

"You'll help me with it?" I feel like I'm back to Square One in some ways. "if when we get closer, if I do want to have sex with him…"

"You're afraid of how you could react to the whole thing. If you'll separate from yourself? Dissociate?"

"I don't think I would. But what if…"

"Then we'd work on it. Right? We'll talk about it as much as you need to…And tell *him*, too. He sounds like he wants to go at your pace."

No one should *have* to die a virgin, I suppose.

Kissing this man is like no other feeling in the world.

Well.
I was prepared for almost *anything* but this.
We were fine.
I was fine.
"We made love last night…." Strauss listens closely. "And I was…absolutely okay…" more and more. "It stayed very… real." I smile. I don't know. I want to think…. I don't know.
"So much…that she's *speechless*!" he teases. And his smile is literally beaming. Okay, okay okay… down fella.
Don't push me!

I don't know where this will go. We're not in some commitment, Jeffrey and I, we just met a while back, this is a romance maybe. With a man unlike anyone I've ever known.
Sorry, Strauss, I know you'd like him to be just an ordinary guy…but he's not.
"Well, *no* one seems ordinary when ya have very strong feelings for them…." Shut up.

Just shut up.
And you're right. But I imagine you already *know* that.

Thursday night.

I'm afraid lately – with Jeffrey. That we'll lose sight of each other, look away for an instant and not recognize the other when we turn back around.

"I'm thinking what if we don't really know each other," I say.

"That you've both been pretending."

"That *nothing* is real..."

"There ya go!" he cries. "Wiping out the whole *universe* rather than be vulnerable to one human being." Okay Okay Okay Okay okay okay okay okay okay okay.

"Ya want to know something?" I say as the session ends. Well, that has traditionally been our pattern. "I could still say exactly what I said the first day I walked in here. With a different meaning, of course." He just smiles and waits. "The world is not at *all* what it once seemed."

One day I might tell Strauss that I'm still half in love with him. Probably always will be. I imagine even Jeffrey knows that. There are times in that session room, even today when I looked in his eyes...there are times...

Not everything must be lost, I guess.

Not as close as I wanted, and not as far as I feared.

I am separate from them – from Strauss, my family, Casey. But I can't be the *concept* of "person" without a history, an imprint. Tainted by others. Or touched by them. Even changed. I will never be a Me who is totally my own.

There aren't even pure properties in physical science anymore. Nothing is sacrosanct, as we now contest every discovery and reinterpret theories from the vantage point of multiple realities. Every ion bumps another, and with that radical Quantum leap, it seems that atoms stay in contact with one another long after parting. Of course, I'd prefer Time and Light to be pure, unencumbered by any matter, unreachable by anything that could be measured or destroyed. Just Time and Light to go on forever, with Matter the mere loser that crumbles and fades. A wave *or* a particle? No. Choose for god's sake. One is right, the other inferior. One is the Answer, one merely an error. Both are. And in most cases, in the deepest of empirical thoughts, we humans simply do not know. "You, your treatment, it's a work in progress, and we'll have to wait and see how it turns out," the smuggest of doctors once said. "And all in all, that's kinda neat." I shrugged off that comment at the time. "It's an adventure!" He'd added, as if that made things more palatable.

We couldn't agree on a lot of our words. Nor could we always make peace to agree to disagree. They can be combat fodder, those pieces of speech. Weapons, sometimes. Rocks thrown hard. Thankfully, we also have gazes -- when we're able to look.

Someone else's eyes seeing back, into us...loving us. If we can let ourselves see.

Of course, those are nothing but human organs. And all in all, rather ordinary.

Eyes that will just die one day and disappear into earth. Nothing lasts.

But memory.